FIGHTING LEUKEMIA AND WINNING

ANTHONY ZAGAMI

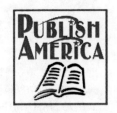

PublishAmerica
Baltimore

First printing

PublishAmerica has allowed this work to remain exactly as the author intended, verbatim, without editorial input.

Softcover 9781627095914
PUBLISHED BY PUBLISHAMERICA, LLLP
www.publishamerica.com
Baltimore

Printed in the United States of America

In the beginning, life can be fine. You grow up happy and in good health. Life can be patient, where you have no worries and things can go tremendously smoothly. Life can be sure for a time, where you are very confident with yourself. Then suddenly it can all change. How do we live life? Do we walk a fine line—watch what we eat, stay away from hazards for fear of illness or death? Or do we live life to the fullest, with no cares or worries, seeking the thrills of a lifetime? After an almost fatal ordeal, you tend to see things differently and appreciate the world; it's a fascinating place to live in, with so much to see and accomplish.

The truth is, we don't really know about life. It's only through the experiences we have in it that we become more knowledgeable. I believe it's not the experience, but what we learn from our experience that counts. I've had some big challenges in my life. Instead of saying problems, I'd rather say challenges, as it makes me feel I have something to beat. It gives more of a positive outlook. Positive outlook can help in any situation. It helps your mind help your body. I use words all the time to change my attitude about things. You can develop a positive mindset through the words you use. Vice versa, you can develop a negative mindset the same way, with words like depressed, destroyed, disgusted, broken-hearted, frustrated, frightened, need help, can't and why me…just to name a few. Consider instead: I will, I am confident things will be all right, great, powerful, strong, winners never quit. I would write quotes in my journal all the time, things I would say not just because of the predicament I was in, but phrases I had used half my life: "winners never quit and quitters never win; I choose to be a winner." Or "life's a journey where the strong survive and the weak perish." And my own, "we live for tomorrow." Think about it.

Never feel guilty about yourself, as most of the time it's not your fault things happen. Sometimes we do make mistakes. When we do, it's best to confess. Life is full of changes. One day you feel happy, as if nothing can go wrong. We enjoy family vacations, fancy cars, restaurants, going to parties, and meeting people. We have hopes, inspirations, plans, and goals. All of these make for a happy life and hope for the future. I am not the smartest guy in the world—far from it—but I always try to use my brain and think things out. It's easy to solve most problems with logic. Example: if you are in a relationship with someone and it's not working out, you realize the best thing to do is end it, even though it is hard and feelings are going to be hurt. In time, the hurt passes and you learn from the experience, just as you know a broken limb will heal in time and is mostly forgotten in time. It's harder to deal with serious unexpected experiences. You tend to realize what's important in life. Financial problems can always be a worry for people, although most people bring them on by spending too much on things that just bring temporary happiness. When you're sick, these things are no longer important and you realize family, friends and people who care about you are the gifts that help you through the ordeal. It's funny how the things you once thought were so important to you at one time—money, cars, jewelry—all seem trivial when you don't have your health.

I am a believer. That is, I believe in God. Not just because of the situation I had been in, but for most of my life. But whether you believe or not, there's something about prayer. I believe that prayer can change almost anything. I don't know if it's mind over matter, but something happens. I've always believed in God, and always will. I never blamed Him for what happened as I believe things happen for a reason and a purpose. My wife believes that the Lord did it so that more people will learn about this disease. I, for one, didn't know what I had until it was explained to me. Not many people know about leukemia, which is a blood disease. It's normally treated with chemotherapy, but in acute cases a bone marrow transplant is the only cure. Who knew what a bone marrow transplant was? I certainly didn't, and I would guess that most people in society didn't know much about the subject either. Unless it happened to a person close to you, you may never need to know. I have seen and heard many stories of people who were in desperate need for a transplant and just couldn't find a donor. The one's who survive, because they found a donor, are few. If more people were aware of testing for bone marrow matching, which is a simple swab of the gum, the chances of finding a donor would be so much higher.

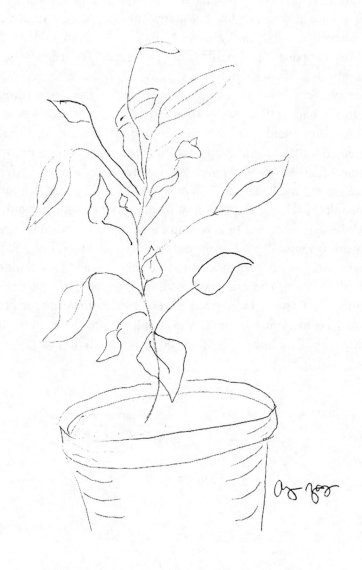

CHAPTER 1

She Opens Her Heart to a Stranger

There's a story that was sent to me from Florida. It became surprising to me that so many people in the world love to give. The woman's name is Lanise Dee. The story was written December 14th, 2006 by Sarah Langdon. She opens her heart to a stranger. Eight years after she signs up to be a bone marrow donor, a woman gets her chance to help. The blood that pumps through Lanise Dees arms is gold—not in color, but in meaning. As she sits, connected by both arms to a machine that separates blood-forming cells from the rest, Dee is at ease knowing that the 60-year-old woman dying of leukemia might live because of this act. Actually, Dee is unabashedly sure that her gift of gold will save this stranger. "I told the bank my blood is a gift of gold. I'm very cocky about my blood," says Dee of Winter Springs. When the regular blood donor signed her name to the national marrow donors program and promised to help if the call came, she didn't realize she would wait 8 years for the phone to ring. But when it did in July, excitement filled her. "I can be at the blood bank in ten minutes," she told the person at the other end of the line. "Give us an hour," the caller responded. That call was indicative of Dee's commitment to just about anything, even cutting her vacation short during the next four months in order to save a woman she knew nothing about, aside from age and disease.

"I assumed someone was ill and I didn't want to delay," says Dee, a mother of three and a grandmother of two. "A delay could mean death. God forbid I ever need it, but I hope someone out there would do the same for me." The need is great. A bone marrow transplant can save those diagnosed with blood diseases such as Hodgkins, leukemia and lymphoma. The transplant replaces unhealthy blood cells with the donor's healthy blood cells, either from the bone marrow, the blood stream or the umbilical cord. According to the national marrow donor program, in the past, blood-forming cells were always taken from the bone marrow, as indicated by the national groups name, in a somewhat painful surgical procedure, typically from the pelvic bone. But more and more doctors are able to bypass surgery and collect the cells from the blood stream with the help of a drug called filgrastim, which increases the number of blood cells in the blood stream. Finding a match could be difficult though. About 70% of patients who contact the N.M.D.P need a transplant from someone unrelated to them, the organization says. Though Dee is one of more than 6 million potential donors on the registry, the group estimates it coordinates transplants for only about 220 patients each month. Dee was only the Florida blood center's 10th eligible donor of that year. There also is the need for ethnic minorities to become donors because tissue type is inherited, just like hair and eye color—meaning someone of the same race and ethnicity will likely be the best hope for a match, the organization says. Dee tells it like it is and has vowed to add at least 100 people to the N.M.D.P. in the coming year. She calls it swab parties; it's a donation where you know where 100% of the donation is going. And you're saving a life. What better can you do in this world? The wait is over. An hour after Dee took the phone call, she gave 9 vials of blood; 2 teaspoons apiece were pulled from her veins. Then she waited for months. "I thought no answer meant a match. I thought, 'how rude they didn't even call to tell me.'" But, in October, when she finally landed at the airport in Dallas, the registry finally called her back. "Had I known, I would have canceled my vacation," she remembers thinking to herself. "I panicked. Do I have to fly home? They told me to relax." When she returned, 20 vials of blood were drained from her body in two sittings, and Dee was to undergo psychological testing to assess how she would feel if the recipient died. Days later she was declared healthy as a horse. For 5 consecutive days she would receive injections to increase the number of stem cells in the blood stream. She was told to expect flu-like symptoms, but all she suffered from was a slight headache. Dee did experience a strange sensation, which she said was feeling her connective tissue as she moved. Finally, on the 5th day in late October, it was time for the donation. Dee sat back as blood from an arm was channeled through a machine and then returned to her body. The process, minus the injections, is the same as donating platelets. It was done during two sessions of several hours, over two days. Dee will receive quarterly updates on her recipient for the first year. Then they will be able to learn each other's identity if both agrees. Dee has signed a release, but she says she'll understand if the other woman chooses privacy. "It would just be wonderful to know she is happy and healthy," Dee says, "I don't expect a thank you. I just wish the best for her." At home, she slowly watches the growth of her plant, given to her by the blood bank as a thank you. "I feel like if I take care of it and it survives, then she's okay," Dee says.

These days, the transfusion for stem cells is mostly done through your arm and not through your hip bone, so the procedure isn't very painful. They do it intravenously through the veins in your arms. In the passage it also says that on her first visit to the hospital, Dee gave 9 vials of blood. A vial is a small test tube that holds about a teaspoon of liquid. That adds up to about half a pint. The procedure takes less than 20 minutes. The whole transfusion lasts for about 2 hours a day, for 2 days. So, first they check you for your blood type, to see how much you match with your patient. Usually like in my case you have to be at least 9 out of 10. But there can be 10 out of 10. The process is an in-and-out procedure. I guess what I'm trying to say is that it isn't that much of an inconvenience to save someone's life.

CHAPTER 2

North Shore Hospital

North Shore Hospital on Long Island, New York. That's where I would live for the next 6 months. Leukemia and lymphoma patients stayed on the seventh floor. There were about 22 rooms, and about 2 patients to a room some rooms were meant to be singles, but all had been full. My stays in hospitals had been scarce and I normally would avoid them— and doctors—as much as possible. In the early 90s, I had an injury to my hand. I was bitten by a pit bull terrier. The bite went right through my hand and broke the pinky bone. I had to stay in the hospital for about a week due to the germs that can get into your bones. Like I said, broken bones heal in time. When I first visited North Shore, I had the same mindset; I figured I'd have a little break from work and I would be back to the same routine that I normally had. Boy was I wrong. Let's face it (or I should probably say, let me face it): I had something really wrong with me and I didn't realize it. I thought I would be back to work in two weeks. Throughout my life, I was always health conscious, always ate right, plenty of fruits and vegetables and exercise. I figured I did the fundamental things that are supposed to help you avoid serious illness, so who would have thought something like this would happen? I guess cancer isn't prejudiced. It'll take anyone.

During my stay in the hospital, I met a lot of people: nurses, patients, doctors, cleaners…all great people…all dedicated to their jobs. Even the patients were. You see, even when you're being treated, you have a job to do. Your job is to get better. I listened to the specialists, assumed they knew what they were doing, and stuck to the daily regimen. Of course there were the medications, but you also have to eat, which most of the time is difficult when you're on chemotherapy. And then, believe it or not, there is exercise you have to do. They suggest walking. So walking I did. This is all part of the therapy.

We walked, my mother and I. We would walk every day. I would walk so often, we would start calculating how far we had walked. Of course, we couldn't leave the floor. And we didn't have to anyway. North Shore is a pretty big hospital. We figured four times around the halls was equivalent to a little less than a football field. I would walk twice a day, even when I was feeling sick, which was pretty often. I was attached to an intravenous drip, so I would have to drag a pole along with me.

Mom's a great woman. Her name is Mary. She was there for me every day. She gave me all the support I needed and the confidence that I could do this. She is a very spiritual person. She studies Yoga and Thai-chi, another great form of stress relief in helping to keep a positive attitude. Walking the halls was how I met most of my neighbors. There was Dom and Francis Bello, Sal D'Angelo, Bill with the bronchitis, a very young girl named Jackie, and Jose. They're just a few of the people I came to know well. Dom was a really nice guy, an elderly man in his late 50s. He knew a lot about blood diseases and blood counts, so I would get a lot of information. He must have been dealing with this situation for a while now. He wasn't the patient though; it was his wife Francis.

She had been dealing with lymphoma, another form of blood cancer that damages the lymph nodes. They were a couple that had been together for over 30 years. Dom would stay in the hospital day and night. We were allowed to have relatives stay overnight. He slept on a recliner that didn't look very comfortable. In these situations we have to do what we have to do.

Francis used to walk the halls with her husband and watch TV in the TV room. They were big Yankee fans. I was Mets. We would tease each other about who was best. Then she started having complications, and so did I. They were the usual in our situation, I would have headaches all the time, almost unbearable. My white blood cell counts were at one, platelets were low, blood counts were low, and on top of that, the fevers. They would measure my temperature using the metric system, so the thermometer would read 38 or 39.

I would get really cold. The coldness would chill right down my backbone, then I would get the shakes. I would shake and shiver so much that my teeth would start to chatter. That's when I knew the fevers were coming, and come they would. All night the fevers were there. I would be cold one minute and then burning up the next. I'd get so hot that I needed ice bags all over my body—my chest, my head, and under my arms. It had become a nightly routine. I remember one morning I felt the coldness and the shaking. I got frustrated. I got mad. I told myself, I'm not going to take this anymore. I'm going to walk. So I did. I walked. And I felt better. The fever was still there, but it was less. I remember talking to Dom and Francis that morning and telling them about the fevers. Francis said, "Yeah, I know how you feel. You have to put the ice all over you and then you sweat 'til the sheets are soaking wet. Then you end up changing sheets all night." I told her I just got up and started walking. Then we started talking about the blood counts and the chemotherapy, both of us waiting for some kind of change.

My roommate at the time was an older man in his 70s. He looked older than that. He looked old. I forget his name. He was there for only a few days. I remember he didn't eat very much, so they would give him a bunch of that Ensure stuff, and the cans would be all over. Anyway, I remember the Doctors coming into the room and telling him his blood counts were up, and the next day his wife came into the room with a wheelchair, wheeled him out the door, and he was gone.

The bed didn't stay empty for long though. The next day, my new roommate was Bill. I didn't know his last name, but I got to know him as "Bill with the Bronchitis." I had nothing against him. I had nothing against anyone in the hospital. After all, we were all there for the same reason: we were sick. He coughed and coughed all the time, and spit out phlegm into a cup. He had also contracted leukemia somewhere, somehow, who knows. He was about my age. I became afraid that I would catch something from all the coughing. I wanted to get out of that room. We would share the same bathroom and all that came between us was a curtain—that was it. I had a fever for days. My temperature stayed level at about 102. I finally told the intern about Bill and complained about the coughing. I remember her telling me, "well, if we were in a perfect world, we might be able to do something." She was studying to be a doctor. She would come to see me every morning at about 7am and give me a check up—blood pressure, heart, lungs—and question me about my diarrhea, nausea, headaches, and so on. I liked her. She was new and still needed a lot of experience. I think it's a tough job taking care of sick people and having to sometimes see them pass away. But I was persistent, so I took my complaint to the head nurse, another great person who really was dedicated to her work. Audrey got me into a different room. I didn't care where I went, as long as my roommate didn't cough. Pretty picky, huh? If you're ever in a situation like I was, complaining a little, don't just sit back. I think it was the right thing to do at the time. They put me in a room with a guy who I called the Redman. He had a rash all over his body. He would joke about it all the time. He used to say he felt like a pepperoni pizza, but really he didn't talk much. To tell you the truth, I wasn't in much of a talkative mood myself. Still, I was happy to be in a room without any coughing.

After a while, my fevers developed into pneumonia. I had it for about 10 days. I didn't remember much about those days. Half the time I was out of it. I remember people saying they came to see me, and I just couldn't place it. I had to rely on oxygen to breathe for a few days. I believe I caught it from the coughing and germs in my previous room. Since I was inexperienced with spending time in a hospital, I didn't know any better. But now I do. Wear protection. Wear a mask. It could save your life.

Francis wasn't doing much better. I didn't know what complications she had. But I think they had to change her chemo. I found that it's not just one type; there's all different types. The next time I saw her, she was receiving oxygen. She still talked and still tried to walk around in her room. I was able to disconnect the oxygen tube and walk the halls. She seemed like she was going to be okay. I talked to Dom. He told me she was having problems. From then on, I noticed she started sleeping a lot and her door was closed most of the time. One morning, while I was walking, I passed her room and this time the door was open. Dom was on one knee, rubbing

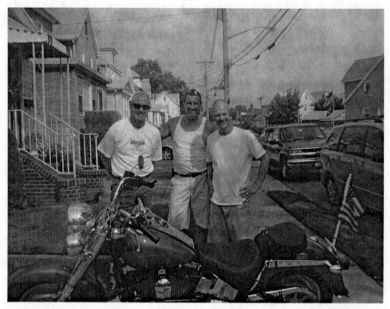

my brother Steve center and a friend Kenny Murphy

Francis's stomach. Well, I just kept walking and thought she must have had another bad night. I later found out that he was saying goodbye. That afternoon I took my routine walk. The cleaners were there, the sheets were off the bed, and she was gone. "Where is she?" I asked in surprise. One said she went up stairs. The other said she went home. But one of them finally said, "She went to heaven." That was my first encounter with death from this disease. Seeing someone die from this brought a little more reality to what I was facing. I think the staff at the hospital is not supposed to mention the patients dying, especially to other patients. It definitely affects your attitude. I couldn't believe it. I saw death from this fatal disease, this germ that creeps into your blood and tries as hard as it can to take you. Now I knew I was fighting something real and powerful.

They eventually moved the Redman to another room and I inherited a new roommate. His name was Jose. Jose was younger than I was. A young man in his 30s. I think he was originally from Ecuador. His story was like mine in that he put off the disease. He didn't want to believe he had it. He let it go for months, started losing weight and then finally passed out one day. I believe he was in another room before coming to mine. He was already on chemo and would often have coughing spells. I wore my mask all the time, even when I slept. He was in the hospital for a long time, about as long as I was, if not longer. I remember he had two sisters who used to visit him all the time. I believe they used to all live together and Jose was the main provider. That's probably one of the main reasons he had put off seeing a doctor for so long. Anyway, they couldn't get it out of him. They kept changing him from room to room. The doctors let me go home for seven days, just to take a break. When I got back, Jose was still there. I remember that when I walked, Jose liked to sit on the window ledge and just stare outside for hours. I knew what he was thinking: if I could just get this thing out of me, I could finally go home.

When I returned to the hospital, this time I was given my own room—703, the same one that Francis had been in. Jose's was right next to mine. By mistake, one day he came into my room, thinking it was his. That day he was very happy because he was finally going to get his bone marrow transplant. He would say, "I'm going to do it, I'm going to beat this thing," raising his hands in the air and thanking the Lord. He was to receive the bone marrow from one of his sisters who matched his blood type. I knew he still had leukemia cells in him, and found it funny that they were still going to go through with it. I also knew that when you did get to that stage, they give you one more shot with the chemo, and hopefully that would do it. I was hoping for the best for him and his sisters, and couldn't wait 'til it was my turn. After he went into the bone marrow transplant room, I never saw him again. I found out months later that he passed away due to complications of the heart. My mom and wife knew, but felt it was better not to tell me.

The first person that I remember seeing on the 7th floor was a young girl in her 20s named Jackie. I felt sorry for her. She was so young and too pretty to be in such a situation. As usual, I'd walk the halls and always stop by to see how she was. Her mom would always talk to me and she really did her studying—checked out all the doctors and hospitals. She always gave me or my mom some kind of advice. Whether it was good or bad, who knew, but we tried anything and everything. I'll tell you one thing: she was always there for her daughter. And who wouldn't be when you're watching your own child suffer. Her mother and father would bring tons of food for her every night, mostly Italian food— eggplant parmesan, spaghetti, pizza. They'd let us eat whatever we wanted at that stage in time. The catch was, you had to have an appetite. Her family would also come every night. Her sister, who was about a year older than she was and in college, and her boyfriend were there all the time. I'd see her father in the TV room and we'd watch the games together. Jackie was in and out of the hospital while I was there and they'd always be surprised to see me every time they came back. Either they were surprised to see that I was still alive, or not cured yet. Who knows? But I know her mother had faith in me and always told me that I'd make it. I never found out what happened to her. The last time I saw them was at the cancer clinic, months later.

CHAPTER 3

Friends

Do you have friends? Is it good to have friends or just acquaintances? Just close enough to say hello when you walk by at work or in your neighborhood? Do you keep to yourself with your wife and family, and keep the door closed? Through my illness I found out a lot about people and friends. Mostly I found out about my family. I think now it's so important to have good friends and family. My father brought us up right. We were proud of who we were and weren't afraid to tell anyone how we felt. He brought us up to be honest and to respect the words of the Bible. It's really just about doing the right thing. We have all achieved a lot together. My brothers and sisters were all there to see me at the hospital. The support felt good. With the situation I was in, I needed all the help I could get. It gives you inspiration. What happened was, I started to realize that you're not just doing it for yourself, but also for your friends and family. I felt they still wanted me around. They still needed me in their life. And my friends made me feel the same. Though some really surprised me. It seemed the friends I thought I knew, I didn't. And the friends I wasn't really close to, were really caring.

It was strange. Before my life changed so drastically, I had friends. Running partners, guys I used to ride with. What I mean by riding is riding motorcycles. I've been riding most of my life. I used to ride my bike to work every day. I started to meet other people on the job. That's how I met my so-called friend. We pretty much hit it off. Liked the same baseball team. Same politics. I was in the Army, he was in the Army. So we had a lot in common. He had known me well. He even went to my wedding. One time, we rode to Lake George, in upstate New York, for a huge motorcycle rally. I think you get the picture. He had moved to a different job, but we still stayed in touch. Sometimes in life, if you don't see each other at the same place, you tend to lose touch. We still talked, but not as frequently. We hung out once in a while. So I found it very odd that when I got my diagnosis my friend disappeared. You would think a person that close to me would come visit and show a little support. I remember talking to him once and I think I was the one who made the phone call. But he did call me once while I was home prepping for my bone marrow transplant. It was November 7th and the reason was to tell me that he was going to run the NYC marathon. I didn't answer the phone; I had caller ID so I knew it was him. Running a marathon is tough, but I think my challenge was ten times harder. Maybe it's the word cancer; maybe they hear the big C word and just run like it's contagious. I have in-laws (more than just In-laws because I've known them all my life, we went to the same schools, and even dated) from whom I got no phone calls, no emails, no cards. So go figure. Then there are friends who I wouldn't have thought would be as caring and concerned as they were. There was John and Darlene Ross, Ken Murphy, Mike Lauri, Will Baez, Lillian, Cathy Zagami and mi wife, and the list goes on. John and Darlene are longtime friends. We grew up together. While I was in the hospital, they would visit me quite often. Darlene was one of my running partners. We ran a Virginia marathon together and also the NYC marathon a few times. I went to school with

John in the 70s but he moved to New Jersey and I hadn't seen him in about 20 years. To me it was surprising how we met again. I was running a race in Central Park. I think it was a 10K—that's about 6 miles. It was a hot summer day. The race was for some kind of charity. Back then, I never really noticed, but the runs were always for some kind of cause like colon cancer or breast cancer. Hopefully I'll be out there running for a cure again. There are about one to two thousand people who run these races. When I finished, I turned in my chip—that's what you tie to your shoe in order to record your time when you finish. After that, I took off my running shoes (I already had my shirt off) and went underneath a hose that was set up to cool you down after the race. Suddenly, I heard a voice call my name. "Anthony, Anthony Zagami?" It was John, whom I hadn't seen in about 20 years. Time does fly, and the world really is small. He looked the same. His wife was running the race also. From there, we stayed in touch and became really close. Then there's my friend Mario, another runner and a really good guy. He runs about 6 minute miles. He was fast. He'd come visit me and bring a pizza or something, and we would go into the TV room to watch TV and talk. I miss pizza at the stage I'm in right now; I'm not allowed to eat anything from the outside. No restaurants, Burger King, McDonalds, Chinese food, none of it. You have to be careful of infections. I have to do this for one year. Then there are the guys at the job. When you're not working and you have a mortgage to pay and other bills, food, kids…it gets tough financially. These guys collected money. They didn't have to do anything, but they collected almost 2 thousand dollars for me. My colleagues went to donate blood for me at the hospital and even had a bone marrow drive; about a hundred people showed up. That was a great turn out. So there are people out there who really want to give. Maybe one day they'll get called to donate for someone else. It would be great to save someone's life. You could become a hero. If you know someone who happens to have any kind of cancer, give support. Be a friend. Get friends to be a friend. I think it inspires a person. I began thinking, "Hey, I'm not in this alone. I'm doing this for me, my family and my friends." Friends 'til the end.

CHAPTER 4

Emotions in Motion

During my stay in the hospital, I had been on various types of medications. Most I took very well. Of course, you know about the chemo. And the side effects that come with it. You are going to get nauseous, vomit, and maybe get headaches, fever, diarrhea, constipation, even sores in your throat. The truth of the matter is that the reactions depend on the drug or drugs being used, and can vary greatly. Even people in the same treatment program can react quite differently. Some people experience few side effects, while others can experience them all. The most common side effects occur in the areas of the body where there is rapid cell turnover such as the bone marrow, hair follicles and the lining of the gastrointestinal tract. Because of these effects, the doctors will issue different types of drugs to help cope with these discomforts. One of the drugs that was subscribed to me was a drug called marinol. Marinol, I found out, is made from marijuana. It comes in a pill. You don't smoke it. It's said that the THC is taken out of it, so you don't get a high from the drug. I didn't think so. I had strange reactions. I felt paranoid. I had weird feelings in the hospital room, seeing people all around me staring just gave me an odd feeling. The prescription did the job though. My stomach was fine and I ate well. I guess it gave me the munchies. I ate everything, all the hospital food—the spaghetti and meatballs, the vegetables, the cakes, all of it. My friends would bring me pizza and sandwiches and I ate it. I had a very good appetite. There was also another effect that the marinol had on me and that was the dreams and illusions I would have. I'd see weird faces in the clouds outside my window. I would close my eyes and not really be asleep, but I would see giant skull creatures like the ones in *Lord of the Rings*. I would think about the leukemia and think of it not as just cancerous cells but as the skull creatures and I'd fight them with my Samurai sword. As soon as I would cut them, they would explode into dust.

Then there were the dreams. Most I didn't remember. But one I remembered vividly. I was in Manhattan, crossing Park Avenue. The thing about it was that I was in my pajamas and had my pole with the liquid medications on it. As I was crossing, a woman in a big white car surged out and almost hit me. I responded by giving her the finger. At that time I was looking for a second opinion on my illness, so maybe I was heading for Sloan Kettering Hospital in NYC, one of the most well-known hospitals in the world. After crossing, I went for my car, a 1991 Ford Explorer. I found my old truck parked somewhere along the side streets, on 71st or 72nd. The door was hard to open, as if it was frozen shut. Finally, I made my way in. It started up fine, but the steering was bad. It was hard for me to drive. I couldn't stop; the brakes were low. I drove up the block and had to make a U turn. As I made the turn there was an old looking candy store with old green paint, big windows, newspapers in front, and rows of candy along the front counter. Inside was my 4th grade teacher, Sister Tarsisius. She had long curly red hair and always wore her black vail. She looked at me and smiled. I kept driving. I finally arrived at the hospital. I tried to park in the hospital parking lot, but they told me that it was full. I turned and went back to North Shore. I got off the marinol. It made me too intense. I couldn't think properly. One of the best tools you have in this fight with cancer is having a positive attitude and I knew that if I stayed on the marinol I would have a lot of negative experiences. Not to mention, right from the start, when you find out you have cancer you become very emotional; you develop a different state of mind. Then you start thinking, "What do I do now? And how do I get out of it?" And about a hundred other questions. From there, you're in your own world—a very different world than you were used to.

CHAPTER 5

Dealing With Chemotherapy

Some people say that dealing with chemotherapy is worse than the cancer itself. It's a tough thing to deal with. I had four bouts with chemo. Each one was different, some doses more potent than others. All with different side effects, as I mentioned in the last chapter. You get nausea, throat sores, constipation, and so on. Oh, and don't forget your hair; it falls out. I picked up a good book from the U.S. Department of Health and Human Resources called *Eating Hints for Cancer Patients Before, During and After Treatment.*

You won't be able to avoid all the symptoms. There are still some you will get. In this book are helpful hints for the discomforts your body feels. If you're nauseous and lose your appetite, you will get medication for it, but with this book you'll know what to eat and what not to eat. Loss of appetite or poor appetite is one of the most common problems that occurs with cancer and its treatments. No one knows exactly what causes loss of appetite. It may be caused by the treatment or the cancer itself.

Emotions such as fear or depression can also take away a person's appetite. Ask a nurse or social worker about ways to lesson this emotional difficulty. Sometimes it's the side effects of the treatment, such as nausea, vomiting or changes in a food's taste or smell that makes a person feel like not eating. If this is the case, work with a doctor or nurse to get the side effects under better control. For some people, loss of appetite happens just for a day or two, and for others it's an ongoing concern. Whatever the reason, here are some suggestions that might work:

— Try liquid powder meal replacements, such as instant breakfasts, during times when it's hard for you to eat solid food.

— Try frequent small meals throughout the day rather than four big ones. It may be easier to eat that way and you won't get full.

— Keep snacks within easy reach, so you can have something whenever you feel like it—cheese, crackers, muffins, ice cream, peanut butter, fruit, and pudding are all good possibilities. Take a small snack when you go out, such as peanut butter crackers or small boxes of raisins.

SORE MOUTH AND SORE THROAT

Mouth sores, tender gums and sore throat or esophagus often result from radiation therapy and chemotherapy or infection. If you have a sore mouth or gums, see a doctor to be sure the soreness is a treatment side effect and not an unrelated dental problem. The doctor may be able to give you something for mouth and throat pain. Your dentist can also give you tips for the care of your mouth. Certain foods will irritate an already tender mouth and make chewing and swallowing difficult.

Try soft foods that are easy to chew and swallow, such as milkshakes, bananas, apple sauce and other soft foods like peaches, apricots, watermelon, cottage cheese, yogurt, mashed potatoes, and noodles. Avoid foods or liquids that can irritate your mouth. This includes tomato sauce or juice, and spicy or salty foods.

DRY MOUTH

Chemotherapy and radiation therapy in the head or neck area can reduce the flow of saliva and cause dry mouth. When this happens, foods are harder to swallow. Dry mouth can also change the way food tastes. Some of these ideas for sore mouth and sore throat may help:

— Have a sip of water every few minutes to help you swallow and talk more easily. Consider carrying a small bottle of water with you so that you always have some handy.
— Try very sweet or tart foods and beverages, such as lemonade. These foods may help your mouth make more saliva.

DENTAL AND GUM PROBLEMS

Cancer and cancer treatments can cause tooth decay and other problems to your gums and teeth. For example, radiation to the gums and mouth can affect your salivary glands, making your mouth dry and increasing your risk of cavities. If you eat sweets a lot you may need to brush your teeth more often. Here are some other ideas for preventing dental problems.

— Be sure to tell your Doctor of any dental problems you have.
— Use a soft toothbrush; ask your doctor, nurse or dentist to suggest a special toothbrush and/or toothpaste if your gums are very sensitive.
— Rinse your mouth with warm water when your gums or mouth are sore.

CHANGED SENSE OF TASTE AND SMELL

Your sense of taste and smell may change during your illness or treatment. Foods such as meat and high protein foods can begin to have a bitter or metallic taste. Many foods will have less taste. Chemotherapy, radiation therapy, or the cancer itself may cause these problems. Dental problems can also change the way food tastes.

— Choose and prepare foods that look and smell good to you.

— If red meat tastes or smells strange to you, try chicken, turkey, eggs, dairy products or mild-tasting fish instead.

— Try tart foods, such as oranges or lemonade, which may have more taste. Tart lemon custard might taste good and will also provide needed proteins and calories. (If you have a sore mouth or throat, tart or citrus foods might cause pain and discomfort.)

NAUSEA

Nausea, with or without vomiting, is a common effect of surgery, chemotherapy, radiation therapy, and biological therapy. The disease itself or other conditions unrelated to your cancer or treatment may be the cause of your nausea. Some people have nausea or vomiting right after treatment. Many people never experience nausea. For those who do, nausea goes away once the treatment is completed. Also, there are new drugs that can effectively control the side effect.

Try foods that are easy on your stomach, such as:

— Toast, crackers, pretzels
— Yogurt
— Sherbet
— Angel food cake
— Cream of wheat, rice, oatmeal

— Potatoes, rice or noodles
— Skinless chicken that is baked or cooked, but not fried
— Canned peaches or other soft, bland fruits and vegetables
— Clear liquids
— Ice chips
— Carbonated drinks
Avoid foods that:
— are fatty, greasy, or fried
— are very sweet, such as candy, cookies, or cake
— are spicy or hot
— have strong odors

Eat before you get hungry, because hunger can make feelings of nausea stronger.

VOMITING

Vomiting may follow nausea and may be brought on by treatment, food, gas in the stomach or bowel, or motion. In some people, certain associations or surroundings, such as hospitals, may cause vomiting. As with nausea, some people have vomiting right after treatment, while others don't have it until a day or two after treatment. If vomiting is severe or lasts for more than a day or two, contact your doctor. He/she may want to give you an antiemetic medication to control nausea or vomiting. Very often you can control nausea and prevent vomiting. At times though, you may not be able to prevent either. Relaxation exercise or meditation may help you. These usually involve deep concentration and can be done almost anywhere. If vomiting does occur, try these suggestions to help prevent further episodes.
— Do not eat or drink anything until you have the vomiting under control.

— Once the vomiting is under control, try small amounts of clean liquids such as water or bouillon.

DIARRHEA

Diarrhea may have several causes, including chemotherapy, radiation therapy to the abdomen, infection, food sensitivities, and emotional upset. Work with your doctors to identify the cause of your diarrhea so that it can be successfully treated.

During diarrhea, food passes quickly through the bowel before your body has a chance to absorb enough vitamins, minerals and water. This may cause dehydration, which means that your body does not have enough water to work well. Long term or severe diarrhea may cause problems, so contact your doctor if the diarrhea is severe or lasts for more than a couple of days. Here are some ideas for coping with diarrhea:

— Drink plenty of fluids to replenish what you lose with diarrhea

— Eat small amounts of food through the day instead of 3 large meals.

Eat plenty of foods and liquids that contain sodium and potassium, two important minerals that help your body work properly. These minerals are often lost during diarrhea. Good high sodium liquids include bouillon or fat free broth. Foods high in potassium that don't cause diarrhea include bananas, peaches and apricot nectar, and boiled or mashed potatoes. Sport drinks contain both sodium and potassium and have easily absorbable forms of carbohydrates.

Try these foods:

— Yogurt

— Rice noodles or potatoes

— Farina or cream of wheat

— Eggs

— Smooth peanut butter with bread
— Canned peaches and well-cooked vegetables
— Skinless chicken or turkey
— Lean beef or broiled fish
Avoid:
— Greasy or fried foods (makes diarrhea worse)
— Raw vegetables and skins, seeds, string fibers or unpeeled fruits
— High fiber vegetables such as broccoli, corn, dried beans, cabbage, peas, and cauliflower
— Very hot or cold food and drinks (drink liquids at room temp)
— Foods or drinks that contain caffeine, such as coffee, some sodas and chocolate
— If you have a sudden short them attack if diarrhea for the next 12 to 14 hours this lets your bowel rest and replace the important fluids lost during diarrhea make sure your doctor or nurse knows about the problem
— Milk or milk products, use sparingly (the lactose they contain can make diarrhea worse); most people can handle small amounts (about half a cup) of milk or milk products

CONSTIPATION
Some anti-cancer drugs and other drugs, such as pain medicine, may cause constipation. The problem is a lack of fluid or fiber, or if you've been in bed for a long time. Here are some suggestions for preventing and treating constipation:
— Drink plenty of liquids, at least eight 8oz glasses everyday—this will help keep your stool soft.

— Get some exercise everyday; talk to your doctors or physical therapist about the amount and type of exercise that's right for you.

— If these suggestions don't work, ask your doctor about medicine to ease constipation.

FATIGUE AND DEPRESSION

All methods of cancer treatments are powerful and may go on for weeks or months. It may even cause more illness and discomfort than the disease. Many patients say they feel exhausted and depressed and unable to concentrate. Fatigue during cancer treatment can be related to a number of causes: not eating, inactivity, low blood counts, depression, poor sight, and side effects of medicine. It is important for you to raise the issue with your health care team if you are having fatigue. Together you can decide what's causing the problem, and many of the causes can be treated.

Fatigue and depression aren't eating problems in and of themselves, but they can affect your interest in food and your ability to stop and prepare healthy meals. Here are suggestions that can help:

— Talk about your feelings and your fears; being open about your emotions can make them seem more manageable. Consider talking with your nurse or social worker who can help you find ways to lessen your worries and fears.

— Become familiar with your treatment, possible side effects, and ways of coping; being knowledgeable will help you feel more in control, so don't be afraid to talk with your doctor and ask questions

— Make sure you get enough rest

— Take several naps or rest breaks during the day; plan your day to include rest breaks

— Make rest time special—reading a good book in a comfortable chair or watching a favorite movie with a friend

CHAPTER 6

How it All Started

To tell you the truth, I don't know how it all started. I think that the biggest mystery of the disease is how you contract it. There are plenty of assumptions, such as smoking, or being close to fumes and gases, but no one really knows for sure.

For me, it didn't happen all at once. There were small signs. I had been living my normal life. Going to work, doing my daily exercise, which was running. At that time I was training for the Long Island Marathon, so I was pushing myself a little harder than usual. I was running 30 to 40 miles a week. At this point, I should have been at the peak of my performance. But I wasn't feeling that way. I knew something was wrong. It wasn't fun anymore. My workouts on the treadmill and the 10-mile runs were getting difficult for me. I wasn't running at my normal pace. I thought, "Well, maybe I'm overdoing it."

I developed a bloodspot in my left eye. I figured it would go away after awhile and didn't see a doctor. It was late March, 2006. I kept going to work and running and I believed the symptoms would pass and I would be myself again. The marathon was in May. I felt myself getting weaker. I would get dizzy spells, and get out of breath easily.

May 7th, 2006 was the day of the marathon and I was registered to run. Marathon Day was here. Guess what: I ran it. Was it hard? Well, a marathon is hard as it is. So doing it in my condition was basically murder, or should I say suicide. Luckily, for me, this course was mostly flat.

It was a great day for a marathon. The weather was between 65 and 70. A clear day. I didn't mind the heat much. I was comfortable running in it. I felt good that morning. I was ready to hit the pavement. Mario was there too. He was going to run the half. He told me I looked like I was ready. Well, we all lined up and were ready to run. The gun fired and we were off. I remember running the first 3 miles and had to stop. But I still had 23 miles to go. I slowed down my pace. I started following a couple of slower runners to adjust my pace. The only problem with that was that I was in race mode and didn't like getting passed much. So I sped past them and thought I was traveling at a great pace, but couldn't keep it up. I had to slow down my pace. I ran another 3 miles but had to stop again. As I was into my next 3 miles, I came across a familiar face; it was my friend from work, Domingo Perez. I don't think I ever mentioned Domingo before, but Domingo was the one who got me started running races. Back in 2002 I ran my first race in Queens. A 5k. I didn't know he was going to be there at the time. Anyway, he passed me by. Still, I forged ahead and made it to ten miles. Then I was coming close to the 13 mile mark. I was hurting. I was weak. I really thought about throwing in the towel, giving up. I said to myself, "I'll just do the half and call it a day." I got to the halfway marker and was about to make the right turn, but couldn't do it. I would have forfeited my goal. In my mind, I would have given up. I would have quit, and my philosophy is "winners never quit and quitters never win." Most of the runners took the right. Then it was just scatters of people left. I remember there was a Korean man running next to me. He said, "We're crazy, aren't we?" I said, "Yeah, you're right." From there, we were on the expressway so all you could see was the open highway and the tree line on both sides. At another time, it would have been a great run. But at that point in time I decided to take it really easy and just enjoy the view. I knew I wasn't going to break my own personal record, so I took out my walkman and just eased on down the road. I would run a mile, then walk about a quarter, then run again, and so on. I had some Johnny Cash, Elton, Billy Joel, and some of my wife's Latin music, at least I had company.

I finally finished at a time of 4:37, about an hour off my regular time. The main thing was that I survived. My wife was worried about me because I was so late. She's very emotional that way. Now that I think about it, I'm surprised I finished in the condition I was in. I ran a whole marathon with leukemia. Today is April 27th, 2007 and the furthest I can run is a half mile. Hopefully that will change.

After the marathon, I still continued working, and not running much, but still running a bit. And still no doctor. My next adventure was a trip with my bro to Laconia, New Hampshire. One of the hobbies I enjoy is motorcycle riding. I started at a very young age. Every year I would arrange a trip either with my brother, friends from work or my wife. The road trips are really fun. I've been to many. There's Daytona bike week, of course, in Florida; Americade, which is in Lake George; and there's Laconia, New Hampshire, just to name a few. Well, this year we were doing New Hampshire. From New York to Laconia, New Hampshire is about a 300 mile ride. I left with a couple of friends from work—James Smith and Mike Rivera. We met up in the early morning, around 6am, and hit the highway. The weather was nice and sunny and I have to admit that I felt good. Once you get past the city

limits, the scenery is beautiful. The trees, the winding roads
and the mountain views are breathtaking. We spent the whole
day riding and we finally arrived at our destination at around
5pm. Don't ask me how I did it, but I did. It was a long ride.
I guess it was the adrenaline that was going through me that
kept me up. I did seem to notice one problem: my hands and
fingers got numb. Other than that, I felt pretty strong. Once
there, we checked into our rooms. I always go to the same
place, The Barry Pond Hotel. We unpacked our stuff and soon
after that my brother Steve arrived. Soon we were back on our
bikes and hitting the town of Laconia. In town there are just
thousands of motorcycles everywhere. Riders come from all
over the U.S. and a lot from Canada too. I would say it's like
a Mardigras type of atmosphere, with bands all over, tents set
up selling bike parts and motorcycles, and let's not forget the
pretty women in their biker outfits. Anyway, we had a good
night. I did try running, as I always did a good 5 or 6 mile run
in the morning to start the day. I got up early, got about a mile
and a half into it, but got tired and had to stop and rest. I turned
around, went back to my room and went back to bed. Well
anyway, I spent the rest of the vacation trying to stay upbeat
with the rest of the guys, but in my mind I knew something
was wrong. James and Mike went riding up in the mountains,
but I wasn't up to it. My brother and I stayed in Laconia and
watched the antique motorcycle races, which were exciting
to see. They were mostly old Indian motorcycles. I got back
home on a Thursday, I was still on vacation.

By Saturday, my wife and I were taking a trip of our own to
the local clinic. I wasn't up to it at first. But by then I was pale,
had dizzy spells, and was tired all the time. I remember lying
on the couch, which I rarely do on my day off unless I just
ran a marathon or something. The phone rang and I got up to

answer it, but I had a bad dizzy spell and almost fainted. Nubia dragged me to the clinic and I remember saying to her, "If there are a lot of people there, I'm not staying." Surprisingly, there weren't. The nurse noticed my complexion right away. I still had the spot in my eye. She said, "You look kind of pale," even though she had never seen me before. After that, she took a little blood from my finger. From that, they noticed that my white blood count was very high. The next thing we knew, the doctor comes in and tells me to go to the hospital. Then he looked at Nubia and said, "Promise me you'll take him to the emergency room right away." Nubia promised.

So we drove to the Long Island Jewish Hospital in Nassau. I signed my name on their clipboard and just sat there, waiting. We waited for about a total of 45 minutes, which I know isn't that much time, but there was something about that hospital that my wife didn't like. Nubia called her sister Martha and told her where we were. She advised us to leave and go to North Shore. North Shore took me right away. They hooked me up to an IV and placed me in a room on the emergency level. Checked all my vital signs and held me there for about an hour, then gave me a room on the 4th floor. They weren't sure what my problem was, but had a feeling of what it could be. By then, my mom was there, and some of Nubia's family. I remember them all standing around the bed and we were all joking about one thing or another. Then a nurse came in and asked if they would leave, except for Mom and Nubia. I will never forget when the doctor came in and told us the news. The doctor's name was Hanna Helinski. When she walked in the room, her face was very serious—as if she had just seen a ghost. She said, "It looks like you have leukemia." Right away, my wife started crying. I still didn't believe it. And besides, I didn't even know what leukemia was. My mom didn't show much emotion. That helped for some reason; it kept me calm. After all, I don't think you would want a bunch of people standing around you crying. I would think that would've made things a lot worse. I still had confidence though. Like I said, I didn't know much about the disease at the time, but I believed I didn't have it. The only sure way of knowing was through a bone marrow biopsy. What's a bone marrow biopsy? A B.M.B is a test that's done on your bone marrow, obviously. But the procedure they use is the hard part. They insert about an inch and a half needle into your pelvic bone. If you feel the small of your back, those two bumps on either side, well that's where the needle goes. The needle is strong enough and wide enough to break through the bone by twisting and turning process. The next day I had my first of many bone marrow biopsies. And that's when I met my regular doctor, Dr. Savanna Well the test results were positive. I had acute myelogenous leukemia.

CHAPTER 7

What's Leukemia?

Leukemia results from acquired genetic damage to the DNA of a developing cell in the bone marrow. The effects are uncontrolled, exaggerated growth and accumulation of cells called "leukemic blasts" which 1) failed to function as normal blood cells, and 2) block production of normal marrow cells, leading to a deficiency of red blood cells (anemia) of platelets (thrombocytopenia) and normal white blood cells, especially neutrophills in the blood. Leukemia cells look somewhat like blood cells. However, the process of their formation is incomplete. When leukemia is diagnosed, the quantity of normal, healthy blood cells is insufficient.

(Acquired from Cephalonia Oncology and Shim Kin Foundation)

Let me tell you my definition of leukemia. Leukemia is a creature, the monster that's in your closet, under the bed when you're a kid, and it finally gets out! It doesn't care how old you are—2 years 5, 9, 21, 43 or 70. It gets into your blood and then tries to eat you alive! And not just you. It's the little girl or boy who hasn't yet had a chance to live life…No Disney World, no rollercoaster ride, no beach on a sunny day. How about a baseball game, or even playing baseball? Or just living a normal life with their family? Once it's in your blood, it doesn't rest. In the months ahead, it eats your liver, kidneys and, finally, your heart.

CHAPTER 8

What to Do?

I kept a journal of every day I spent in the hospital. It helps remembering names of doctors (you see a lot of them), names of medications, and just some things you do throughout the day. Here are some excerpts from my journal in the first few days in the hospital:

6/17—Emergency room at North Shore Hospital. Blood work pointed to Leukemia. Low platelets, low red blood cells. High white cells. Received 2 pints of blood a positive.

6/19—Operation was done for bone marrow and blood, 8:30am. Results in 2 to 3 days. My heart examination was done while waiting for results.

I guess they were checking my heart because taking chemotherapy has a strong effect on it.

6/20—Interventions in collarbone, three-pronged should last 14 to 21 days. Chromosomes should show how long the treatment will last. In the next few days, should start chemo.

The three-pronged intravenous in my collarbone was called a catheter. A doctor inserts a small tube either in the neck or underneath the collarbone. The tube goes directly to your heart. As it says in the journal, it lasts for 14 to 21 days. My first one was inserted on the top of my collarbone, so it was on my neck. You can have problems with it if it isn't inserted correctly. It can get infected and cause fevers. That's what happened to me. One of the reasons why I was getting fevers was because the catheters weren't inserted correctly. This happened not once, but twice. The third time I finally got it done right; they inserted the catheter, but this time they used a sonogram machine, which is something like what's used to look at a baby in the mothers womb. I had no problems with it for the rest of my stay in the hospital. A suggestion, if you are ever in a predicament like I was: tell the doctor you would like to get it done with a sonogram.

Now I had a new companion: a six-foot pole with a meter on it. Wherever I went, the pole went with me. I'd walk the halls with the pole in my hand. In my room, when I slept. Pretty much always. I had its decorations too—sodium chloride, sometimes bags of blood if not blood platelets, and of course the famous chemo.

The chemo looked like any of the other bags of medications. It wasn't green and glowing. And it didn't stand out from all the rest. But the effects were phenomenal. The liquid would infiltrate your system a drop at a time, for days at a time.

Besides having to drag the pole around with you, it would also malfunction a lot. When something went wrong, the machine would start beeping. And so you would have to contact the nurse every time it malfunctioned. Pretty much the whole day you would hear beeping noises from the machines. I remember when I would take a shower, my nurse would disconnect me from my pole and tape up the hoses coming out of my neck so they wouldn't get wet. Well, I was so used to having my pole on wheels that I would take it with me anyway, until I realized I was disconnected. It was pretty funny.

My room number was 711. I thought it was a lucky number since my daughter Caitlin's birthday was on that day. It wasn't as lucky as I thought. That was my first room, on the 7th floor, where I met my friend Bill with the bronchitis. You know the rest.

My children, Candice and Caitlin, were very concerned at this point in time. They had always looked at me as a strong father who was able to handle anything. When they saw me in a hospital bed with pajamas on and an IV pole, it was clearly going to be a tough fight. They didn't say much, but they knew it was a life or death situation.

I remember sitting down with them and telling them that they would see me go through a lot of changes due to the effects of the chemotherapy. I said, you're going to see me lose a lot of weight, and also my hair is going to fall out. Some days you will see me sick and vomiting. I figured I'd let them know in advance, before they started to see my body deteriorate. I also told them that we would get through this and that it was all part of the procedure in curing my cancer. I said this with a tear in my eye. Because, like I said, I was always strong and I think they never believed that something like this could happen to their father. Well, cancer isn't prejudiced; it goes after anyone.

I wanted to stay alive to see my children grow, and to care for them. Slowly you begin to believe that it's not just for you anymore. You do it for your family, friends and especially for your children. I knew I had a tough fight ahead of me, but was determined to win. I started walking the halls and even got an exercise bike in my room. I rode the bike twice a day. I thought that through exercise and the sweat and burning of energy, I would make the good cells stronger and have more of a chance to kill the bad cells. I would eat as much as I could, take all of my medications, and believed that I would beat this thing.

THE FIGHTER

I fight a battle everyday against discouragement and fear
Some foe stands always in my way
The path ahead is never clear
I must forever be on guard, against the doubts that sulk along
I get ahead by fighting hard
But fighting keeps my spirit strong
I hear the croaking of despair, the dark predictions of the week
I find myself pursued with care, no matter what the end I seek
My victories are small and few, it matters not how hard I strive
Each day my fight begins anew, but fighting keeps my hopes alive
My dreams are spoiled by circumstance
My plans are spoiled by fate or luck
Some hour perhaps will bring my chance
But that great hour has never struck
My progress has been slow and hard
I had to climb and crawl and swim
Fighting for each stubborn yard, but I have kept in fighting trim
I have to fight my doubts away and be on guard against my fears
The feeble croaking of dismay has been familiar through the days
My deepest plans keep going wrong
Events combine to thwart my will
But fighting keeps my spirit strong
And I am undefeated still!

This Poem was a gift to me while I was in the hospital from my mother's friend Terry. It fits.

CHAPTER 9

Yes, Things Started Happening

As I said earlier, my stays in a hospital had been very rare. So I didn't know what was going on and exactly how serious my condition was. It seemed like they had given me every test in the book. I had my heart checked, CAT scans, and they checked the level of my breathing and my blood every day. This was all new to me. It seemed like I had attracted a lot of attention—everyone was watching me.

My friends from work would come visit me, like Mike Lauri, and just give me that look, like I feel for you and hope you can make it. And I told him, "Why the look? Don't worry, I'll be OK." I also told him to tell my friends not to visit. I didn't want visitors at first because I didn't want them to see me in this condition. Also because a lot of people would come and I was weak, my immune system was low, and I'd have a great risk of catching something. They still came and called. I didn't mind.

One of my friends, John Benefonte, a fellow bus driver who we called Murry the Cop because he looks like the cop from *The Odd Couple*, would call me every so often. His son had AML but didn't make it; he died at a very young age. As I got more and more involved with this disease, not by my own choice, I learned more about how many people around me had someone they knew that was affected by cancer. Mostly tales about how, out of nowhere, people would contract this disease and would survive. These are the stories you want to hear, of course.

I was given books to read—plenty of books. One book that I read was written by Lance Armstrong about his battle with cancer. The name of the book is *It's Not About the Bike; My Journey Back to Life.* It was very inspirational. He had testicular cancer and eventually it reached his lungs, then his brain—and he beat it! He had the problem of waiting too long to see a doctor, which I think is one of the most essential things about beating cancer. Well, anyway, I thought that if he could beat all of that then my chances should be pretty good...

There's another story that wasn't written in a book. It's about a man (I only know his first name—Nelson) who is the son-in-law of one of my mother's friends. He had contracted lymphoma and had it bad. It was so bad that most doctors wouldn't see him. The doctors he did see gave him a slim chance. He went from doctor to doctor and each had the same story. Still, he didn't give up. Finally he found a doctor in Texas that helped him and finally cured him. He's been in remission for over six years. And is back to work with the police department. He has also set up a company, through a charity in Texas, that builds homes for cancer patients who have to travel there to undergo the outpatient process of medication and therapy.

Now it's my turn to beat this thing. After three days in the hospital, I got used to the routine. When I had my visit from the intern at 7am, I was ready; I was determined. She would check my lungs with the stethoscope—heavy, strong, deep breaths—and would check my blood pressure, which would pretty much be normal, and would ask me if I had any pain or diarrhea or sores in my throat. Then she'd take a vial of blood and later on, during the day, I'd find out my blood counts.

I felt good. I felt strong. I felt I didn't have much reaction to the chemo. And I even felt that my hair wasn't going to fall out.

Making the rounds that week was a Doctor Bradley. The doctors in the staff would rotate the 7th floor with the interns once a month, and then the next month another doctor would do the rounds. So I didn't know Doctor Bradley very well, considering it was almost the end of June. One thing about him was that he got right to the point and didn't hold back any punches. He told me that, yes, my hair would fall out and that I would be tired and weak, but he did say to go out and walk. I started getting headaches and nausea all the time, but I still rode the stationary bike everyday, no matter how I was feeling. I figured there would be some complications, so I countered through exercise.

EXCERPTS FROM MY JOURNAL

6/21—Treatment started 5:30pm. Alopurnall tablets (1) daunorrubien (chemo) cynosure. Zairian to prevent vomiting.

6/24—changed my nausea sickness pills to marinol 5th day of chemo. Have been taking Tylenol for headaches, still no appetite but still eating regularly. Feel a little better after I eat.

6/28—Day 12. No chemo. Still no effects, still eating fine but did lose 4 pounds looks like I'll have to get a bone marrow transplant in the future, within the next 3 months, will receive more blood and platelets today. Will see bone marrow specialist today (Dr. Bayer) it's a common procedure.

6/29—2nd day off chemo. I feel fine so far, still eating. No new drugs. Jeanette cut my hair. Received more platelets and two bags of blood.

As I was writing in my journal, I started to feel as if I were some kind of mad scientist doing an experiment on myself, turning from Dr. Jekyll to Mr. Hyde. In the journal, I wrote about Jeanette cutting my hair. Jeanette is a friend of mine from my step-daughter Jhoanna's soccer team. Her daughter plays soccer with Jhoanna. Also there's Lillian—I call her Lilly—who also has a daughter on the team. Another good friend of mine with a great heart. These two are always together. Anyway, I figured I'd cut all my hair off before it fell out. She cut it like a crew cut, not totally bald.

7/15—Today should be the day I get my bone marrow biopsy, which should tell me a lot about my progress. Hopefully the bad cells would be gone. B/p 137/86 Temp 36.5 Bicycled for 3.8 miles.

I remember being excited about the outcome of my bone marrow test results. I felt the chemo had done the trick. I had a vision in my head that my doctor would come in and say, "The results of the bone marrow test show no signs of leukemia." I woke very early that morning, in fact I didn't sleep much. I remember talking to Maria the intern and telling her that I didn't sleep much because I was too excited about getting my results.

7/16—Didn't sleep well. I had something on my mind: the test. I have been thinking positive and praying. Just hoping for a speedy recovery. Hopefully we'll have some good news today. B/P 182/82 temp 37

The news wasn't good. That day I got a visit from a doctor who made the morning rounds. Dr. John, a female doctor. She was very pretty and looked like she was from India or from that part of the world. Before she came into my room, I had gotten my regular visit from Maria the intern, the one who checks my vital signs and asks if I have any problems. I remember telling her that I was excited today because today is the day I'll find out my results of my second BMB. If the chemo worked, the bad blood cells would be destroyed, and I'd be able to go home.

Doctor John said that the chemo didn't work. There were still signs of leukemia in my blood. Of course, it was a big letdown. I had always been in good physical health and thought I'd beat this thing with the first dose. After I heard the news, I ate my breakfast, then started walking the halls again. As I walked, I ran into Dr. John again and asked her how many leukemia cells were still in my system and I remember her saying it was a significant amount. Later on that day, I received my first visit from Dr. Bayer, the bone marrow specialist. The next step was to do a bone marrow transplant. We started talking about bone marrow transplants and stem cell transplants and whatever else there was to be done to beat this thing. I needed donors. The best donors possible would be from my family—brothers, sisters, mother, father. In my case, my parents were too old. Then my cousins all started giving their blood to see if they were a match. Nubia and a friend of hers from work, Jennifer, started a bone marrow drive. Nubia worked on having a drive in the bus depot and also in Manhattan. They made flyers and put them in the local areas. The drive went well. My fellow bus drivers who were able to donate, did. Nubia's coworkers also gave.

Jennifer contributes a lot of her time helping cancer patients. After losing a close friend, she ran a marathon far charity. I think she collected 10,000 dollars. I still have yet to meet her. We have shared emails though. And one day I hope to run a race with her.

My two brothers, Steve and Dave, were hoping, as I was, that they would be a match. We weren't lucky; they didn't match. Lorna was next, and from the first vial it seemed like she was the one. It looked like we had a match. She was eager to help. My hopes were high and I was ready to get started. I wanted to get into that bone marrow transplant room. I remember being in the TV room and knowing the transplant room was next to it. I wanted to be in there. I had the feeling that that was where I had to be in order to survive. Behind that door was a mystery to me. I had seen people going in and out, but didn't know what was waiting on the other side.

There was a Russian patient who I would always see in the TV room. He worked construction. He was in his late 50s and we would talk about everything. He was very jovial. We talked and joked around a lot. He liked to tease the nurses. He would tell me about life in Russia. He was there until the age of 16 but said he started drinking vodka at 13 because it was so cold there. His visits were pretty much routinely back and forth to the hospital. He was in some type of remission. He was an outpatient, but came in for small doses of chemo. I asked him about the BMT room and he told me that there is nothing to it, they just give you a blood transfusion intravenously. He wished he was able to do it, but he had a weak heart and didn't want to risk it.

At this point in time, we were searching for answers, making phone calls to different hospitals. Everyone we spoke with—that is, Mom, Nubia and friends in the hospital—all knew a good doctor. There was Sloan Kettering, the famous hospital in NYC and just how good North Shore was and the doctors that worked there.

Mom went to the computer and looked up Dr. Savanna and Dr. Bayer and found that they were pretty good at what they did. Also found that North Shore was rated number 5 in the country. Still, we consulted others. There was Doctor Gabby

Love, who was recommended by one of Nubia's friends, located at Columbia University Hospital...Dr. Markowitz at Sloan Kettering...a Dr. Neil Cohan at the Carl and Dorothy Bennett Cancer Center in Connecticut...a Dr. Schuster at NY Presbyterian (Dr. Schuster started the bone marrow treatment at North Shore, then went to NYP)...then there is the famous Dr. Applebaum in Seattle.

I thought it over. Made a few phone calls. But being so far into the procedure here and having to send out all of my medical papers to another hospital would have made things that much more difficult for me. I was close to home at North Shore, so I decided to stay.

Things didn't change for the better. My health didn't change. In fact, things had gotten worse. Things weren't going as I thought they would be in my mind. By now, I thought I'd be home. I had accepted the fact that my first bout with the chemo didn't work, but from there things started getting worse. I developed pneumonia. I had headaches and fevers. I went for a brain scan and as I was going back to my floor I looked at the results. I thought I read that they had found something, that I had a tumor in my brain. Don't know how I read it, but thank God I was wrong. The results were negative. On the 7th of July I started my second round of chemotherapy. Hopefully, this time, it would kill all the bad blood cells in me.

Excerpts From My Journal

7/7—Didn't sleep well last night. Had a bad day, felt cold, had a headache all day. I threw up in the morning. I'm going to ask to switch rooms; too many people in this room could be susceptible to infection. Had to take a sleeping pill last two nights in a row, received platelets, running high fever. Second dose of chemo. Daunorobicine for 5 days.

7/9—3ʳᵈ day of chemo. Still have a fever, it's been going up and down. Received blood yesterday—2 bags. The first pint made me dizzy and had a paranoid effect. Got up to go to the bathroom and blacked out for a second, thankfully I landed on the bed.

7/12—Slept very well this morning. Rode the bike for a half hour, over 7 miles. Today is the last day of my chemo. Don't know yet if I need blood or platelets. I got some encouraging news today. I found out that a 73-year-old woman was cured by Dr. Bayer, and to make it more significant her son is a friend of mine (Mario). Played piano, Temp normal, 36.9. Received 2 pints of blood. Biked again for 30 min. Took a shower at 7 o'clock.

Mom had made plans earlier in the year, before this all started, to go on vacation with her Thai Chi group to Sedona, Arizona. She was contemplating canceling it. I talked her into going and promised her I would be OK. She had been in the hospital every day. I thought she could use a break, so she left for a week.

During that week, I developed pneumonia. I talked to Mom on the phone in Sedona and told her that everything was going fine. At the time, I didn't realize I had pneumonia, but had a lot of trouble breathing. Before I knew it, I was depending on an oxygen mask to breathe. My mother told me that Arizona was beautiful with the huge rocks and red landscapes. One of the rocks there is a big healing rock. I don't know the name of it, but it's well known. People go there to pray. Mom told the group about my situation and I had 24 Koreans and 6 Americans praying for me at the rock. I believe in prayer; it works.

EXCERPTS FROM MY JOURNAL

7/26—We know what the problem is. I have water in my lungs so I'll be getting medication for that too. I think this is the cause of my high fever. Felt good during the day, played the piano for about an hour. Tried watching the Met game on TV but got tired and went to my room and slept. Caught the ending though—they won.

7/27—Had a fever last night, as usual, about 11pm. They checked my vitals and my temp. Was at 40, took out the cool blanket but this time I didn't sweat as much. My temp did return to normal and hasn't changed since. Was 37 all day. Had a good day, received platelets in the morning, eating good.

7/28—Still having slight fevers. 38, no fevers, no problems with that, but I have water in my lungs which prevents me from breathing properly, had a hard time breathing and sleeping in truth I'd rather have the fevers.

7/29—Today I feel fine. Mom's back and I have more confidence in myself. Will be getting platelets today, blood count is up to 5, B/P 137/84 temp 35, weight 163, injected with neupegen to build white blood cells.

I started receiving neupegen shots to increase the growth of my white blood cells. At this point in time I was getting homesick. I wanted to get this thing over with. I was getting very impatient. It had been 41 days so far in the hospital. I had seen other patients going in and out all the time and they'd come back and say "WOW you're still here" and I'd say "Yeah, I'm still waiting for my counts to go up." It had to reach 7 and no fevers.

8/4—Still having fevers; good news is pneumonia is almost gone. Haven't been writing much, missed a few days. Biked for 20 mins. Walked for 30.

8/6—Day 50. Had a fever at 5 in the morning until about 7. Today they took my portal out, hoping that was the cause of my fever, we'll see tonight. Received platelets.

8/7—No fever last night, should have a good day today. I got platelets and 2 pints of blood.

As you notice, in the excerpts I was going through a lot of blood and platelets. Don't know where it all went, but I was glad it was there for me. I had a lot of donors, a lot from my job. If they couldn't see me, at least they could give me blood. All the nurses in the blood donor clinic knew my name by heart. I'm sorry I can't do the same for them; after a bout with cancer, you are not able to donate blood anymore.

8/8—No fever last night. I had the bone marrow test, the results are for tomorrow.

8/11—Report on bone marrow test showed still signs of leukemia cells, so I'll need more chemo. Doctor says they can't use his own stem cells for the transplant so hopefully one of his siblings will be a match. Platelet count is still low and potassium count is still low. Gets shots of neupegen to boost white blood cells.

When I wasn't up to writing, mom would write in my journal:

8/12—Sleeping well every night, counts are going up. Doctor Savanna was here today. He told me what the next procedure would be. We will be taking high dosages of chemotherapy for 6 days, 2 times for 3 hours every day—this should knock out the rest of the leukemia. Then we go directly to the bone marrow transplant.

Dr. Savanna was the first doctor of Oncology that I met in the Hospital. He gave me a positive attitude about this whole ordeal. He told me that he'd get me better, back on the bus and running again. Dr. Savanna looked like a doctor. He had dark black hair, parted on the side, round rimmed glasses, a mustache, and usually wore a 3-piece suit under his white coat. He liked buses. Don't know why—he did have a car. It seemed to me that he had taken bus rides often. He liked the fact that I was a bus driver. I don't know if it was to take my mind off of things for a while or just to be inquisitive. Anyway, I told him about the bus route I was doing at the time. I drove the Q32, a bus route that goes from Northern Boulevard in Queens all the way to Penn Station in Manhattan, via 5th Avenue. He told me that he had taken that bus before. You actually drive by a lot of famous sites—over the 59th Street Bridge, down 5th Avenue past St. Patrick's Cathedral, the Empire State Building and then finish at Penn Station in front of Madison Square Garden. It's kind of a busy line, but you get used to it. I've been driving a bus for 14 years now. Hopefully I'll be back soon.

CHAPTER 10

You Don't Know What You've Got 'Til You Lose It

The chemotherapy did kill a sufficient amount of the cancer cells, but not all of them. There was maybe about half left in my blood. In order to get a bone marrow transplant, you have to be totally free of the cancer cells, so my second try wasn't good enough. Well, I hope it's not like baseball—3 strikes and you're out.

The doctors decided to send me home. I really needed it. After all, I was in North Shore for two months. They filled me up with blood and platelets before I left, and I had an appointment at the outpatient clinic the next day, but at least I would be home.

As you can imagine, I couldn't wait to get out of there. I was up early, took a shower and changed into civilian clothes instead of the pajamas I wore in the hospital. We waited until about 3pm until we finally left. As soon as I walked out of the hospital, I felt great. It was a beautiful day. It felt good breathing the fresh air and seeing regular people just walking and living life. I noticed everything. I saw everything in a different way. The trees, the sky, the clouds…it all looked fresh and new to me.

I remember crossing the Whitestone Bridge and seeing the boats and the water. It was beautiful. I felt free again. When I finally got home, the house looked great. It was still the same—no changes really—but to me, everything looked great, better than ever. I missed my home, and sleeping in my own bed again was just incredible. You don't know what you got 'til you lose it.

Well, we didn't waste any time. We did everything after we left the clinic, where I had to get even more platelets. We went out to eat at one of my favorite places, the Outback Steak House. I had a steak and the blooming onions. What a difference from the hospital food.

The next day, I was up early again and, believe it or not, I went for a run. I ran and walked about a mile. Later on that day, I went to my job. It was good to see my old friends. A lot of them didn't recognize me because I was bald and had lost a lot of weight. We talked and joked around of course. When I left, I told them I'd be back in February.

The following day, I was back at the outpatient clinic for more platelets. After that, with Dr. Savanna's approval, we went to the NYC aquarium with the kids. On the 18th of August, Nubia and I went to Jones Beach. On the 19th I received more platelets and blood. After that we went to the movies to see *Pirates of the Caribbean* and on Sunday we had a family BBQ in the backyard.

August 21st it was back to the hospital. This time it was room 712—a single room, no roommate. The chemo was to start the next day. I had my heart checked and everything was OK. My weight was pretty good—165, 15 pounds off my normal weight, but I did gain 15 pounds on my 7-day leave.

We started the chemo, as planned. It was called cytarabine. 2 times, 3 hours a day. This stuff was strong. I lost my appetite. I was nauseous and vomiting all the time, and also had diarrhea. This chemo also had an effect on your eyes, so I had to take eye drops 3 times a day.

On the 30th of August they decided to change my room. They told me that someone was in need of it more than I was. I didn't put up a fight. I left quietly. I went to room 707. It was a two-person room. It was the last room at the end of the hallway. The room was cold; there was a constant wind from the air conditioner that came in from the ceiling in the hallway. It felt like it was about 50 degrees in that room. You would think it would be simple, just close the door. Well, the guy who shared the room with me wanted it open. I developed a fever within hours. I remember lying in bed, covered with two blankets over my head. The cold felt like it was going right down my spine. I was just laying there, shivering. Finally, I got up and walked to the front desk and told them I wanted out of that room. My counts were low and couldn't handle the constant draft. The nurses actually saw my teeth chattering as I was talking and felt for me. I entered that room at 3 and left at 7 the same day. I lay in the TV room while I was waiting for another room, still shaking and shivering for about 2 hours more until I was finally moved. My new room was 703—Francis's old room. It was a single room and it was big. I remember the walls being red. It was a big, red room. I thought about Francis when she was there and I hoped that I didn't leave the same way she did.

CHAPTER 11

The Day My Wife Saved My Life

It was September 1ˢᵗ 2006—my second day in my new room. I had been carrying a slight fever all day. I didn't think much of it, seeing as lately I always had a high temperature. We were watching TV. She usually would bring me a small piece of cake and a coffee for a snack at night. But that night I didn't feel like it. I wasn't feeling well and so we went back to the room. As soon as I got there, I threw up. Usually at this time, around 8:00 in the evening, Nubia would make her way back to the house with the kids, but tonight she had been reluctant to leave. I lay in the bed slowly, starting to fall asleep. The fever was getting higher and higher. It got to 105. I was sweating and I felt like I was in a daze. The nurse that I had was new and it seemed like she didn't know what to do. Nubia told her to get some ice packs. I didn't want them, I just wanted to sleep. My wife made me put them all over my body, under my arms, on my head and on my stomach. It's a terrible feeling. I could feel my heart beating rapidly and my breathing was very heavy. Nubia kept dousing me with ice packs, and by then the doctor was there. He was a young Asian doctor who I guess worked the night shift. He told me that my heart was beating very fast. I said, "I know, I can feel it." They loaded me with sodium chloride water. There were about three huge bags on my pole because my blood pressure was so low—80 over 40. I really felt out of it, as if I was in another world. Then they came with the X-ray machines, I struggled just to sit up.

Nubia stayed with me in the hospital the whole night. I looked up at the clock and it was only 11:00 at night, but I felt that with everything that happened it seemed a lot longer. They say time flies when you're having fun. Well, I guess I wasn't having much that night. My heartbeat didn't slow and my blood pressure still stayed low. I couldn't sleep. I didn't feel like sleeping anymore. I stayed up the rest of the night and just tried to relax myself. If ever I thought I was going to die, I think it was that night. If my wife wasn't with me that night, I think things would have been a lot different. The next morning I said to my wife, "Honey, you saved my life last night."

CHAPTER 12

Still No Changes

EXCERPTS FROM MY JOURNAL

9/1—High fever during the night—105, diarrhea returned. Dr. Hersch found infection in blood; received two pints of blood and one bag of platelets. Can't eat, keep throwing up.

Dr. Hersch was my infection doctor. He was the one who helped me with my pneumonia. Since my bout with pneumonia, Dr. Hersch visited me regularly. I liked him. Usually he'd bring good news. Like, your lungs are clear from pneumonia and your white blood counts are going up. That was always, and still is, good news. I was still having slight fevers on September 11th—I was sent down for a pulmonary test. That's when you blow into a tube as hard as you can to check your breathing. As I did, I felt air rush up to my left ear and got swelling behind my left ear. It was pretty painful.

9/14—Still have swelling in my left ear, will be taking X-rays today. Dr. Hersch explained to me that the lump was called Mastoiditis and prescribed antibiotics. He said when my blood cells went up it would disappear.

As you know, my bone marrow transplant doctor was Dr. Bayer. At this point in time, Dr. Bayer and I didn't see eye-to-eye. She knew then how I was feeling. You see, she's been doing this for a long time. At this point in time, things weren't going well for me. My doctor was still Dr. Savanna. He came to my room at least once a week to see how I was doing and would explain to me just what was going on. Bayer would make the rounds almost every day. She didn't give much attention to me. She'd pass by every once in a while and ask how I was feeling. She'd mention a thing or two about the transplant, but not in very much detail. I was curious. I wanted to know about the transplant. I wanted to learn everything about it.

I didn't know then what I know now. Dr. Bayer has a lot of patients. She goes from the hospital at North Shore to the outpatient clinic, taking care of patients. It must be a very busy schedule. By the way, she drives a PT Cruiser convertible.

I was going through tough times. Like I said, I wanted some answers. I wanted to at least hear some good news. I was still coping with my disease, it was still in me. I wanted to find out the answer to this. How do I get it out of me? There were no matches, and my blood counts weren't going up. I took it out on my doctor. I had told the other doctors that I had felt that Dr. Bayer was ignoring me. Dr. Coletz was making the rounds that month. One day he came in with another three interns and I think the head nurse. He asked me the usual questions, taking notes and telling me my counts. In return I told them my list of problems. I remember I had big welts on my head and on the sides of my temples, I had had constipation for days, and one day I had pushed so hard that my eyelids turned black and blue. I had headaches all the time. I had the mastoids, that swelling behind my ear. I told them I wasn't getting any answers from Dr. Bayer about the transplant and I wasn't told anything about my sister being able to assist. Well, somehow it got back to the doctor. The next day, she came into my room, very upset. At the time, I got upset over anything myself. We didn't really know each other—just a couple of meetings in the hallways and very rare visits to my room. I kind of went at it with her. I told her how I felt—that she wasn't giving me much information. I felt that I knew nothing about what was going on and what had to be done. I wanted to know if they had a match for me, and if I even needed a transplant. Would my brothers and sister or cousins help? I was finding out from different sources—other patients, different doctors and anyone who had any info for me. In my mind, I felt Dr. Bayer wasn't paying enough attention to me. In the long run, I found out that at the moment it wasn't my time yet. I wasn't ready for a bone marrow transplant. I still had leukemia. It was then that she told me about my blood counts and not finding a donor. She was right. She had done this before. In order to have a transplant, first there must be no signs of leukemia in your body.

I thought again about switching doctors. It's always good to get a second opinion, even trying different hospitals if you have to. In the end, I stayed with Dr. Bayer.

CHAPTER 13

Padre Pio

I was still getting regular visits from my friends and family who really hung in there with me. Mario, Eddie (Jhoanna's soccer coach), John and Darlene Ross, my cousins John and Linda and Lillian and Jeanette would always come. One day, Lilly came with a book. She took it out of a bag and on the front of it was a picture of a man whose face I had seen before, but I never knew who he was. I finally found out it was Padre Pio. He is a famous man in the cancer world. That's our small world that not many healthy people are aware of. You see, in this world, you hear the stories of the 6-month-old baby who's in desperate need of a donor, or the old man who keeps coming back to the hospital for his chemotherapy treatments pretty much for the rest of his life, and once in a while you hear about a miraculous story of someone who's near death and for some reason or another he or she survives. Lillian is part of that world. She had suffered from breast cancer so much that she told me that if she ever had to go through it again, she would not do it.

I looked at the book and said "Padre Pio?" I looked again and then laughed. The only saints I knew were Saint Francis and the Apostles. She said to me, "Promise me you'll read it. The whole book." The book was about 400 pages. I looked at it, then agreed. What did I have to lose? My counts were down, cancer was still in me, and I couldn't find a donor anywhere in the United States. My brothers and sisters weren't a match. Lorna had come close, but it would have been too much of a risk. She was 7 out of 10. So I read.

The national review called him "The hottest thing in mysticism in the 20th century and one of the chief religious forces in Italy." By 1968, Padre Pio from Pietrelcina, whose secular name was Francisco Forgione, was receiving 5,000 letters a month and thousands of visitors were converging on him from all parts of the earth, making their way through Italy's Garbanzo mountains to the little 16th century Friary of Our Lady of Grace just outside the town of San Giovanni rotunda, near the city of Foggia. There they would wait for days for a chance to make their confessions to him, packing themselves into a friary church to "assist" in Padre Pio's Mass.

Hundreds of books and articles were written about him in his native Italy and scores of stories appeared in other countries as well. *The New York Times, Newsweek* and the *New York Times Magazine* from time to time featured lengthy serious articles about the man who was widely known as the second Saint Francis. At least two Popes said privately that Padre Pio was a saint.

Despite his plump, rosy-cheeked appearance, he was plagued by a variety of physical problems from the very beginning of his novitiate. He suffered from intestinal irritability, as well as attacks of vomiting so intense that he sometimes was unable to retain food for weeks at a time.

Once, for a space of six months, he was forced to subsist largely on milk. He suffered from spasms of violent coughing, was tormented by headaches and frequently ran high temperatures without warning. Pio would seem to be reduced almost to death, only to recover just as suddenly. His superiors, through medical consultations, tried unsuccessfully to pinpoint the cause of his physical troubles.

In 1908, while Pio was studying at the Friary of St Egidio at Montefusco, physicians made a devastating diagnosis. Noting the asthenia, or weakness, of the 21-year-old patient, coupled with the severe respiratory problems and fevers, which were most severe at night, they declared that he was suffering from an active case of tuberculosis of the lungs.

Until 1909, his illness did not prevent his progress toward ordination. Pio received minor orders at Benevento on December 19th, 1908 and two days later ordained to the sub diaconate. The next month, at Marconi, he was ordained to the diaconate. Then he collapsed; his stomach could retain nothing. During this period Pio kept in touch with a Padre Benedetti and his letters from this period show him to have been in very low spirits. He was very depressed by his poor health. In April, he was confined to a bed. In May, he suffered from chest pains. In July, these pains were so bad he was rendered speechless at times. "If the almighty God in his mercy desires to free me from the sufferings of my body, as I hope he does by shortening my exile here on earth," he wrote Benedetti, "I shall die very happy."

Padre Pio liked to identify himself with Simon of Cyrene, the man who was forced to carry the cross to the hill of Calvary after Jesus had collapsed under its weight. Like Simon, Pio did not imagine that he had chosen this mission himself. He was certain he was chosen by God, to be a victim to help carry the cross.

On the afternoon of September 7th 1910, Padre Pio appeared at the high Priest office and showed him what appeared to be puncture wounds in the middle of his hands. He asked him what had happened. Pio told him that he had been praying in the Piano Romania when Jesus and Mary appeared to him and gave him the wounds.

Padre had the Stigmata for the rest of his life. It would come and go. He would wear gloves to mask what would frequently get bloody and stained. Padre Pio took great pains to conceal the wounds. Father Dominic's description, which dates from 1949, describes Padre Pio's practice ever since the appearance of the Stigmata: Padre Pio wears brown gloves [woolen] during the day. These absorb the blood if there should be any and at the same time don't show any. During the night, he frequently wears white gloves, which are sometimes soaked with blood by morning. Padre Pio washes them himself in the sink in his room. Padre Pio washes his feet in the sink in the kitchen, but in the corner so that his wounds are not open to gaze. Regarding the wounds on his side, this also bleeds continually so that he must change those 2 or 3 times a day. The small pieces of cloth are furnished by people around here. These he keeps in place with a band around his chest. In addition to the inconvenience of the persistence of messy wounds that had to be frequently cleaned and dressed, Padre Pio suffered real pain. He frequently replied to those who asked him if the Stigmata hurt, "Do you think the good lord gave me them for decoration?"

Padre Pio's interior life—his prayer, his meditation, his communication with God and the invisible world—was the most important aspect of his existence. It dominated his life of action amidst daily affairs. For most of us, as far as our conscious experience is concerned, prayer is a one-way conversation. We trust that God hears our petitions, accepts our praise and thanksgivings, and pardons our sins, but our senses do not perceive his response. For Padre Pio, prayer was often an emphatically different kind of experience. God literally spoke to him, sometimes through a word perceived through his organ of hearing, sometimes through a vision perceived through his organ of sight, but more often through the vision that is not seen and the voice that is not heard.

There are many accounts of cures and conversations dating from the late 1930s and the early 1990s. In November 1935, Padre Constantine Capobianco became ill. He went to Padre Pio and told him he had been diagnosed with tuberculosis of the lungs and was being ordered to report to a sanitarium in Rome the very next day. This was his second bout with this disease. "Don't worry," Pio reassured him, "this is only an excursion; the Lord intends the same results as the other time." The treatment was successful. Padre Constantine was soon discharged and he outlived Padre Pio.

In 1939, the celebrated Italian comic playwright Luigi Antonelly came to San Giovanni, Rotundo. A short man with thick limbs and a dark moustache, the 57-year-old Antonelli was known for his sweet smile and the light of goodness in his eyes. His need was very great, as he had been recently diagnosed with cancer of the face, neck and jaw. His doctors wanted to operate, but under direct questioning admitted that even with the surgery Antonelli would die within 6 months. The playwright had been about to submit to the operation when a friend told him about Padre Pio. Thereafter, he left his home in Pescara and journeyed to San Giovanni, Rotunda where he attended mass and made confessions to Padre Pio, "I cannot repeat what he said to me," Antonelli recounted, "because while he was speaking to me I seemed to be living in a supernatural world." Antonelli noticed an improvement at once, and soon his cancer was arrested. A few months later he wrote, "I don't know whether the word 'miracle' is correct from a theological point of view, but I will not split hairs about words. I am now writing an article every Sunday for the *Giornale D Italia*. I go hunting. For the past month I have been working on a comedy that will be produced at the Manzoni Music Theater in Milan. I don't know what doctors think about it. I don't know what X-rays and histological examination may reveal. But today I feel that I am cured."

When Antonelli refused surgery, his doctors told him that he would die in 3 months. Yet he survived for 3 years, working and active most of the time. Before he finally succumbed, he told his experiences to another noted author in Argentina, Dino Segre, who wrote under the pen name of Pitigrilli.

Pitigrilli, then 46, was well known in both Italy and South America and by his own admission he was a materialist, though he had been a seeker of the truth for some time. When at Foggia, Antonelli had told him to go to San Giovanni Rotundo, and he did so.

Pitigrilli attended Padre Pio's mass, sitting far back in the church. As far as he could tell, he was completely unknown and unrecognized. To his amazement, during the part of the mass where the priest urges the congregation to pray for various intentions, Padre Pio said, "Pray brethren, pray frequently for someone who is among us today, someone who is in great need of prayer. One day he will approach the Eucharist table and bring many with him who have been in error like himself."

Although not called by name, Pitigrilli was convinced that Padre Pio had him in mind. Feeling as if his heart were bleeding, he dissolved into tears. When he approached Padre Pio for confession, Pio said to him, "What profit a man to gain the whole world and lose his sole, truly God is good to you."

Another South American devotee of Padre Pio was Monsignor Fernando Damiani. Damiani made numerous trips

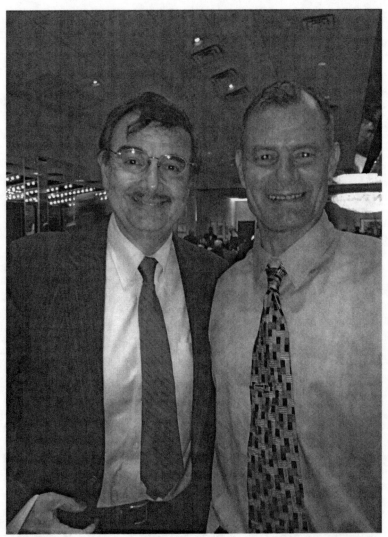

Dr. Savvana

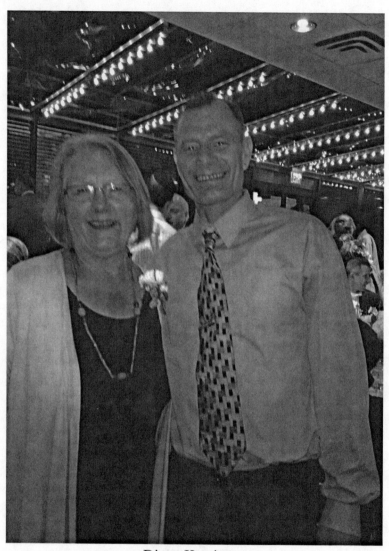

Diane Kessinger

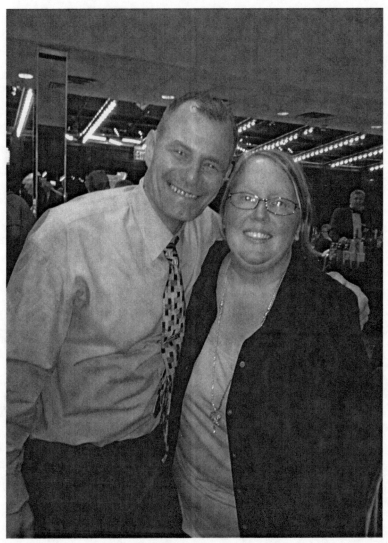

Dr Ruthie–Lu Bayer

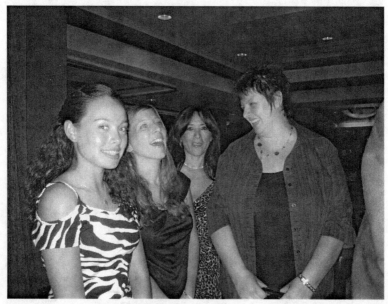

My stepdaugther Jhoanna, the translator, mi wife Nubia and
Martina at the Survivors Dinner

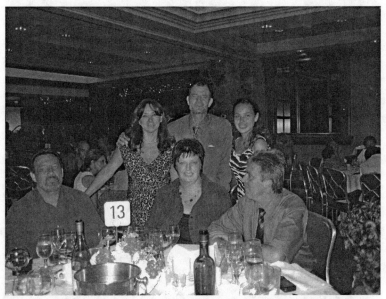

Steve 'Nubia' me' Jhoanna 'Martina' Andreas Martinas
husband.

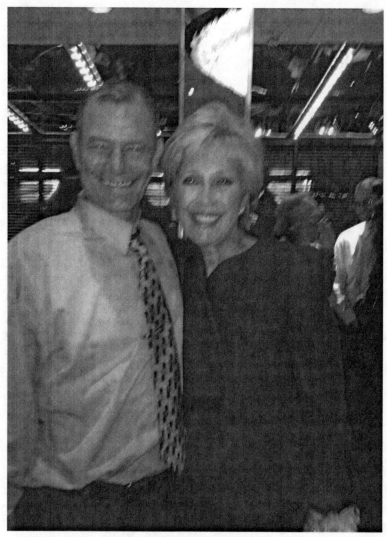

Caroline Monti Saladino

to see Padre Pio…In 1929 the Vicar General was diagnosed with cancer of the rectum, but after prayer by Padre Pio all signs of the malignancy disappeared. Specialists in both Rome and Paris refused to believe that he had ever had cancer until Damiani showed the X-rays taken in Uruguay. When Damiani visited San Giovanni Rotundo in 1937, he was suffering from severe coronary disease and in great pain. He asked not for a cure, but said he had come to San Giovanni to die close to Padre Pio. While at the Friary, he had a major heart attack and lay for hours. At the point of death, he asked for Padre Pio, but to his dismay the friar remained in the confessional and did not come to him until he was through hearing his penitents. "Why didn't you come earlier?" demanded the old prelate, "I could have died already."

"I knew that you would not die," said Padre Pio, very matter of fact, "and so I continued to hear confessions." He told Damiani that he was to die in Uruguay. When he was ready to travel, Damiani should return to Uruguay and continue his ministry.

Damiani stayed up until 11pm talking with Archbishop Barberri. At a little past midnight, Barberri, who had returned to his room, was awakened by a knock at his door. He opened it. The room and the corridor were both dark, but he thought he could make out the form of a man in a capuchin habit. "Go assist Monsignor Damiani," said the friar, "He's dying." The knocking at the Archbishop's door was overheard by a priest by the name of Padre Francisco Navarro, who was awake and praying in the chapel on the same floor. In the meantime, Barberri ran to Damiani's room. The door was unlocked and when he got no response from his knocking he went inside and found Damiani in the throes of another heart attack, speechless and lying across the bed where he writhed, breathless and contorting with pain. Damiani had a little writing table; on it was scattered pills for his angina pectoris, as well as a note written in a faltered hand. It seemed to be scratched or outlined in the form of a telegram: Padre Pio San Giovanni Rotundo. Unrelenting spasms in my heart are destroying me—Damiani had collapsed before sending the telegram.

Opening his eyes and seeing Barberri, Damiani mustered the strength to ask the archbishop to administer his last rights. Running to fetch the necessary materials needed, Barberri awakened everybody around 12:30 in the morning. On September 12, 1961, Fernando Damiani, Vicar General of Salvo, died surrounded in his final hour by four bishops and six other priests! As Padre Pio had promised, he died well assisted.

A few years later, Archbishop Barberri went to San Giovanni and asked to speak privately with Padre Pio. He asked point-blank whether he was the capuchin who passed the door telling him to assist Damiani. Padre Pio gave an evasive answer and the archbishop insisted. Still Pio answered evasively. Then Barberri laughed and said, "ho capito" (I understand). Padre Pio nodded and said, "ha capito" (yes, you understand). Barberri asked Padre Pio to assist him on his death bed, to which Pio responded, "No, I will die before you will, but I will assist you from heaven." Barberri, who lived to be 87, did in fact survive Padre Pio by 11 years.

Pio's only nephew, Ettore Masone (son of his late sister Felicia), also lived for a time in San Giovanni; he had come there after the death of his father in 1940. However, at the end of the war, Ettoruccio, as he was called, returned to Pietrelcina to open a movie theater. When he asked his uncles advice, the padre told him to be careful about the films he showed as you don't want to contribute to the propagation of evil.

Shortly after he opened the theater, Ettoruccio suffered a severe epileptic attack, which was followed by pneumonia, then pleurisy. Maria Pyle, who had gone to Pietrelcina to look after him, phoned Padre Pio to tell him the doctors wanted to operate. "Well, if necessary, let them operate," he said.

Even after surgery, Masone failed to rally and was sent home in a condition worse than ever. Not yet 30, he was resigned to death, telling his friends and relatives to pray not for his recovery but for his soul. Soon he fell into a coma. Some years later, Masone recounted, "I found myself at the gates of heaven, where my sister Giosepina, who had been dead for years, was standing. And then I saw Padre Pio. Both of them wouldn't let me into the gates of heaven."

Meanwhile, Pyle, the physician, and the others in the room were convinced that Ettoruccio was dying. Unconsciously, he cried over and over, "ZIO PIO ZIO PIO!" It was recalled that his mother spoke in a similar fashion before she died. Certain that Ettorucio was about to die, his relatives phoned the church to make funeral arrangements for the next day. No sooner than they hung up, Masone had come to; he shouted, "I'm not dying anymore!" His recovery was complete and instant.

Perhaps the most curious and unusual characteristic of Padre Pio, and the one least able to be explained, is his ability for "dislocation." That is, Padre Pio, while physically in San Giovanni Rotundo and often in full view of his confreres, was nonetheless seen, heard and touched in other parts of Italy, Europe, and the rest of the world.

WHY PADRE PIO?
Why Padre Pio? Why the book? Who was this man? Now that I think about it, I remembered the cleaners with the Padres face on their cleaning carts, and necklaces with his face on

them. And, as far as I could tell, everyone knew who this man was. Some even had stories. Who was this man who is now a saint? And who was alive for only 5 years after I was born? I didn't know, but I read. I would read the book that Lillian gave me every day while I was in the hospital. Nothing miraculous happened. I didn't have visions of the Padre. I didn't start reading and then all of a sudden jump up out of bad and scream, "I'm cured!" But I read and read, and I can tell you this: there were small subtle changes. Positive changes. For one, my blood counts started rising. And I'll tell you, that is a very positive accomplishment. I was feeling better about myself and I had a feeling that, this time, my bone marrow treatment would be negative for leukemia when the time came for it. Also, my temperature was gradually returning to normal.

Meanwhile, there was still the ongoing search for a bone marrow donor. Or did we still need one? My leukemia was generated by bad chromosome cells, which meant that I couldn't have an Antilogous transplant—meaning I wasn't able to do it with my own stem cells. Patients can use their own stem cells depending on their situation and the type of leukemia they have. What happens is, the blood comes out of your arm and is filtered. The filtered blood is then frozen. The patient undergoes chemotherapy. After that's done, they transfer the filtered blood back into the patient's body. And if all goes well, the patient is cured. This type of treatment is called a peripheral blood stem cell transplant. No matter what type of transplant you receive, the cells that are being transplanted are stem cells. These are immature blood that will grow into red blood cells, white blood cells or plasma cells, replacing the cells that have been damaged or destroyed by the disease.

Dr Bayer and Dr. Savanna did come up with a third alternative. They knew my situation and had discussed it between themselves, and decided that I would be able to get what is called a cord transplant. Like bone marrow, umbilical cord blood contains stem cells. It comes from the umbilical cord of newborn babies and is removed from the placenta after, then stored. Once a cord match has been identified through the cord blood registry, the cord blood is then shipped to the Seattle Cancer Care Alliance. This type of transplant, at the time, was done only in two places in the U.S.—Seattle and Cleveland. Not exactly a short drive away. My wife and mother were going to take time off from work and we were all planning on taking a trip to either Cleveland or Seattle. We had gotten in contact with the Seattle Cancer Care Alliance only to find out that my insurance wouldn't cover the procedure. What was the cost? $300,000 for starters. What would you do? After all, it's your life we're talking about. Do you forfeit your house for it? Give up all your material things for your life? Suddenly you realize that that stuff is meaningless. We made phone calls and tried every angle we could think of. Finally we found that the hospital in Cleveland would accept my insurance. I didn't want to go; I really didn't feel up to traveling hundreds of miles. I had been thinking a lot those past few days about traveling that far and having some procedure done on me that I didn't know much about. But I figured, if I have to do it to survive, then I will.

I was still in the hospital, going on 8 weeks, still reading my new book and still hoping for some kind of change, some kind of positive news. I was tired. I was getting weaker due to all the medications, the fevers, the chemo. All of this bad news was finally taking its toll. My attitude was changing. I was tired of this hospital, I was tired of the everyday test and evaluations, and yes tired of the doctors too! I had to get home. I needed a break. It was August 21ˢᵗ 2006 when I finally got some good news: after my fifth bone marrow biopsy, the results showed a negative finding of leukemia! No leukemia cells in my blood. Was it a coincidence? After 3 bouts of chemo. Was it really true? Did the Padre have something to do with it? Who knew for sure? I had faith in the Padre and felt he was with me now. I would read my book every night before I went to bed. The doctors and nurses noticed the book on the side of my bed. It was always there, beside my bed, on the night table. You may think it was corny or just foolish or whatever. I just knew in my heart that something was changing for the better. I would read and pray, and would thank God, Jesus Christ and Padre Pio for being there.

EXCERPTS FROM MY JOURNAL
9/26 B/P—142/90 no fever at 9:30 am. White blood cells up to 3. Got more good news today—we have found two donors in Europe. Hopefully they'll be a match!

I couldn't believe it. I had a real chance of surviving this ordeal and actually living a normal life again. I remember making my daily walks through the halls and thinking about it. Finally someone. A person out of nowhere. A total stranger, willing to spend time and probably some money, going out of their way to help someone they didn't even know. I felt my heart in my throat and shed a tear—maybe more than one. Tears of joy, happiness and gratefulness. On September 29ᵗʰ 2006, I went home, this time free of leukemia. Just a note: the feast day of Padre Pio is September 23ʳᵈ.

The name of the book is *Padre Pio: The True Story*, by C. Bernard Ruffin.

CHAPTER 14

Back Home

I was back home. For how long, I didn't know. Still, it felt good to be back home. It always does. I did my usual thing. I worked around the house as much as I could to get ready for the winter months—putting the lawn furniture away, straightening out the garage—but I was always aware of what I could do and what I couldn't do. My leukemia was gone. I was in remission. Well, I wasn't exactly sure, but I felt I was. Still, I had plenty of medication to take. I always wore a medical mask when I was around people or working in the garage or around dust. I did get out. I got my motorcycle and took it for a ride around town; I did some golfing with my brother (played nine holes at Van Cortlandt Park in the Bronx); and I did my runs, though not far—I would walk and run for about a mile.

I was feeling good—almost like I was back to normal again. We would also go out to the driving range and just hit golf balls. I'd hit about 150. Then, after that, we would get some ice cream and eat it at Cochran Park in Queens. Actually, I was never a golf person until I got my illness. While in the hospital, one of my room had a view of a golf course, so every once in a while I'd just sit and watch the golfers play. I started watching it on TV too, and eventually bought a video game. Then David brought me to the driving range to get my swing down. I figured it wasn't a very tough workout. All you had to do was swing a golf club, right? Try it. It's not as easy as it looks.

Of course, I had my doctor visits. I was still seeing Dr. Savanna. I'd go through my normal routine—get my blood checked, my weight (which at the time was good, 165) and also my blood pressure and temperature. Everything looked good. My white blood cells were good. They were up to 11— that's like a normal person. Everything else was also fine. I did need platelets every so often. We would still talk about the transplant in Seattle. We had found a donor, but who knew if they were willing to subject themselves to the procedure. If you read Chapter One you know what they have to go through.

Still, I went on with my life, not really worried either way, thinking maybe I would not have to do any. Maybe the leukemia was gone for good. Remember, I had Padre Pio on my side. I was prepared for anything, staying in shape as best I could, and I ate a lot; somehow I had a big appetite. I would eat 4 eggs for breakfast, 4 slices of toast, hash browns, bacon and orange juice. Some days it would be oatmeal or cereal with toast. My wife would make arepas on the weekends, which is a Colombian dish made from toasted corn flower and then you put ham and cheese in between with butter of course. For lunch it was hero sandwiches—turkey and roast beef, cheese, lettuce, tomato, and mayo. And sometimes my favorite: chicken cutlet parmesan. For dinner, usually spaghetti and meatballs (usually I'd go for seconds). It was either that or rice and beans with chicken. Sometimes we'd go out for Chinese, Spanish or Italian. I was beefing myself up— first, because I had lost so much weight and second, because I was to be tested again and I wanted to be ready. I remember I would pick up Jhoanna from school and we'd stop and get

Burger King and I'd order a Whopper, fries and a thick shake. Jhoanna got a Junior Whopper with fries and a Coke. It was fun. I felt like a real "cucino"—in other words, a PIG. But I didn't care. I was on a mission. And I was alive again! I had been out of the hospital for three weeks and still no word from my donors.

Meanwhile, I still had my routine checkups. No sign of leukemia, but my counts were gradually going up. WBC count was up to 17. My Hmg was high, and also my reds were normal. I thought that was great. I was feeling excellent and had plenty of energy. Dr. Savanna didn't feel the same way. He had a very serious look on his face; something was wrong. I remember that day I went to the clinic with my brother Steve. He asked if it was good that my counts were going up, and Dr. Savanna said not necessarily. I needed platelets that day and the doctor, as he usually would, walked with me to the appointment desk to arrange for platelets. As we walked together, I asked him if it was possible that I wouldn't need a transplant, that maybe the leukemia would be gone for good this time. He said no, it'll come back. Guess what: as we were walking, the cancer was slowly returning. And he knew it. I didn't have much time left if I didn't find a donor soon or get to Seattle or Cleveland. Everything that I had worked for all these months would have been for nothing.

I started making phone calls again to Seattle and talking to my insurance agent, mainly to a man named Richie Boletti, who really seemed to be concerned for me—not only for my insurance but also for my health. I'd ask him for advice and he would always give it to me—even pharmaceutical help. He'd say, "If you need any help with anything, give me a call," and I would.

Mom, Nubia and I were trying to work out a way to get to Seattle. You see, Seattle had Dr. Applebaum, one of the best in his field. We started making arrangements for tickets online, as well as a place to stay while we were there. We would have to stay there for at least 6 weeks. On top of that, we had to conjure up some money for the trip. We thought of fundraisers like raffles or some kind of fundraising dinner to get there.

Well, on my next visit to the clinic I got some news from Diane. Diane Kissinger was my head nurse whom I would see and speak to often. This time I was with my mother. While we were waiting to see Dr. Bayer, Diane had come out to see us. The news was good. One of the donors had agreed to donate her bone marrow cells. Yes, it was a female. We were all smiles and the jokes started coming—like, maybe after the transplant I'd start doing lady-like things and it would change my sexual appetite. And I'd say, "but you'd still love me anyway, wouldn't you?" Later, we found out that she was from Germany and I would joke about having a craving for kielbasa and knockwurst and that my hair would grow back very dark and I'd grow a moustache right under my nose. Hey, it's all in jest—and by the way, laughing can add eight years to your life and boy could I use that right about now.

Back to being serious. We started talking about the transplant and what had to be done. We went back to the TV room on the 7th floor of North Shore and watched videos of people who had gotten bone marrow transplants and some of their donors. One guy was lucky and his brother was a match; he explained how he felt donating his marrow and claimed that, for about a week, he did feel weak and a little light-headed, but other than that he was fine. His brother had explained what he had gone through on the other side of the transplant.

First, he had planned everything out. He brought his favorite books with him and his laptop computer so that he would be able to get his work done while he was in the quarantine. But he found out while going through the chemo and the transplant that he wasn't able to do anything because he very weak and tired all the time. He did survive though, and I believe he was on his third year of recovery.

The other story I remember was that of a young man, maybe 21 or 23—I've forgotten exactly, but I did notice that his story was similar to mine. They called him TJ and he was in desperate need of a transplant, but could not find a donor. He had been searching for a long time—I think over a year. Like me, he finally found a donor in Europe. I remember he was a light-blonde-haired man and then, after the transplant, he looked totally different. He had really dark hair and grew a beard. If you're interested, you can still see his story on the internet. It's called "A Brand New Life." Look up Fred Hutchinson Cancer Center in Seattle or bone marrow transplants.

TYPES OF TRANSPLANTS
The name that covers all types of blood transplants is Hematopoietic cell transplant. There are three types:

Bone Marrow Transplants.

Peripheral blood stem cell transplants

Cord Transplants

The differences among the three types of transplants have to do with the source of the transplanted cells. In each case, doctors are transplanting stem cells, immature blood cells that are made in the bone marrow. Stem cells grow into mature blood cells of various types. The transplanted cells may come from your own body (an antilogous transplant) or from some other donor (allogeneic transplant). This person may be a related donor (a family member) or an unrelated donor. The type of transplant you receive depends on your situation. The major advantage of an antilogous transplant is that you will not face the complications of Graft vs. Host Disease. However, with an antilogous transplant you also do not have the same Graft vs. Host benefits. As a result, there is a higher relapse rate with antilogous transplants, and this type is not suitable for a number of diseases.

Bone Marrow Transplants—If you have a bone marrow transplant you will receive bone marrow that has been collected from a donor. The donor may come from a family member, or he or she may be an unrelated donor whose tissue type closely resembles yours.

Peripheral Blood Stem Cell Transplants—Stem cells are produced in the bone marrow and circulate in the blood stream. These cells are called Peripheral Blood Stem Cells, or PBSCs. If you have a stem cell transplant you will receive stem cells that have been collected from the blood of a donor who may be you (antilogous transplant) or a sibling or other relative or a closely matched non-related donor (allogeneic transplant). The antilogous stem cell transplant donor may be any age. But the allergenic donor must be older than 12.

Cord Blood Transplants—Like bone marrow transplants, umbilical cord blood contains stem cells. It comes from the umbilical cord of new infants and is removed from the placenta after birth and then stored. Once a cord match is identified through the cord register, the cord blood is then shipped to the patient.

I was to receive a bone marrow transplant. We started talking about the transplant itself and of course there were a lot of questions. The room was called a clean room. It wasn't a sterile room, meaning I would have to stay in a bubble and no one could come in. But it was to be cleaned everyday—floors mopped, walls cleaned and furniture too (which wasn't much), sheets changed, the works. The room itself was only about 10 feet by 10 feet. Just room for a TV, bed, a small writing desk, and a few chairs. I did have a big window where at least you could see the outside world. The thing about this room was, once you went in you couldn't leave until the whole procedure was over, and that was at least 4 to 6 weeks. One more thing: the toilet facilities. It was a portable cameo (meaning a chair with a bucket in the middle) that took a while to get used to. As far as bathing, I used baby wipes and took sponge baths. What's a sponge bath? Well, I'd stand in a tiny 12 x 16-inch plastic tray with a bucket of warm water and just doused myself with soap and water, and wiped myself with a sponge.

After the conversation, Mom, Nubia and I were asked if we would like to see one of the rooms. I know earlier I said I was dying to get in there (literally). But I figured there would be plenty of time to get acquainted to the room once I got there, so I didn't go. Mom and Nubia did, and they didn't have much to say. But they did see a patient that had gotten some type of transplant and had been getting ready to leave and they said that he looked to be in pretty good health. With some transplants you don't even lose your hair.

About the transplant itself: I, as you know, would be getting a bone marrow transplant. The bone marrow would go through my blood stream intravenously, same as if I was receiving regular blood or platelets. Before you are able to receive the new bone marrow, you have to get rid of the old. And yes, you guessed it, more chemotherapy. This time the chemo was called Fludartine Melphalan. I got it for an hour and a half each day, for 7 days. On the 11th of November, 2006, I was back for the third time at North Shore Hospital. I had been out of the hospital for 5 weeks and I didn't miss it. Now my PJs were packed, as well as my tooth brush and my slippers, and I was on my way.

When I arrived at the hospital, I had to register at the administration office. The person registering me had to put me in a wheelchair in order for me to go to the 7th floor. She ended up wheeling me up herself (usually they send an assistant to help). I could have walked, but I guess she was worried. Well, when we got up to the 7th floor, she was so surprised that everyone knew me there, she didn't know that this was my third time at this. The nurses were happy to see me, and they all wished me luck. Then, finally, I was there at The Bone Marrow Transplant Room. This was it and I was ready. I came in with a full head of hair and weighed 179 heavy pounds.

Everything was planned out. The chemotherapy was to start the day of my arrival, and it did. My white blood cell count was at 15.5 and my platelets were 169 (a normal WBC ranges from 3.8 to 10.5). Anyway, with the help from the chemo, we would get it down to 0. That's everything. If you've ever heard the expression "bone dry" well, when the treatment was done, that's what I would be.

The chemo was working well, and this was the first time I was looking forward to seeing my counts go down. To say the least, I was really astounded by how fast the chemo was taking its toll on me. They were really hitting me with some strong stuff this time. Each day my weight was shedding by at least 5lbs. I thought that there had to be something wrong with the scale. I even had them bring another one in. But the scales were correct. By the end of my treatment my weight was down to 141 pounds. And in eight days, my blood counts were down to 0. And, of course, my hair was gone. I was totally bald again. I have to say, I looked like a real cancer patient. I only found out from pictures afterwards. There were no mirrors in the room. All that needed to be done now was the transplant. The bone marrow cells were coming all the way from Germany. My donor had donated the cells the day before, on the 16th of November. They were put on a plane the same day and sent to the U.S and I was to receive them the next morning.

November 16th was a rainy, cold, windy day. It was around 5 in the evening and at this time of year, daylight was gone. We were all just sitting in my room, waiting and talking. I remember the wind pushing against the window pretty hard. I believe it was Mom, my wife, my sister Lorna, and her daughter Lana. We were pretty quiet that night, just watching TV and mom says, "imagine if something happens to the plane while it's on its way and we lose our precious shipment of gold." I had heard a story once of a man who was to receive a heart transplant and the plane went down—with the surgeon who was to perform the operation on board! It was like we were sitting around telling ghost stories. All we could do now was pray and hope everything went well.

The next morning, the sky was bright. The sun was out and everything seemed OK. When Maureen came in with a smile on her face, I knew everything was a go. Maureen was the head nurse at the bone marrow transplant room. By the way, she always seemed too cheery.

On November 17th, 2006 my transplant started. I was to receive my shipment of gold. In the cancer world, they call this day your birthday. I guess because you become alive again; you have a chance to be cured and live a life free of cancer.

The bags looked like regular bags of blood, but much thicker. It took a long time for the stem cells to go through my system. The transplant lasted 5 hours. There was no pain and also I didn't have much of a reaction to my new blood.

I did my normal thing: lie in bed, watch TV, and read. Also, I had my laptop computer. Mostly I'd use it to play video games, Tiger Woods Golf and also a game called Call to Duty, an army war game.

The following day, I felt very weak. I was vomiting and had heartburn. On the third day, my feet and legs were numb and sore. It was a weird feeling—nothing that I had felt before. It was painful at times, almost like having authorities. My face and eyes were swollen and my eyes were also bloodshot. Apparently this was to be expected. For me, the heartburn and the sore throat was what really bothered me. It felt as if my esophagus had gotten smaller. It was hard for me to swallow. I had to take liquid medication 3 times a day for it. Like usual, the headaches came, and the fevers too. Needless to say, there were many sleepless nights. And the nights I slept, the dreams were always there. Usually I didn't remember many, but one I do.

MY DREAM/NIGHTMARE

I had been sleeping comfortably in my 10 by 10 room when, all of a sudden, I was awoken by a loud, almost jack hammer type of banging. Still so weak from my transplant, I didn't feel like getting up to investigate what was going on. Suddenly, two men broke right through the wall, then one climbed out from under my bed. I had to struggle to get up. It was hard for me to move, as I often feel when I dream. I noticed that they had been speaking a foreign language. I asked them what they were doing here. And in turn they told me they were renovating the room. They had power tools; they were sawing down the walls while dust was flying everywhere, and there was this high pitched scratching sound like devils laughing. It was the noise from the sawing. I couldn't handle it any longer. I knew I wasn't supposed to leave the room, but I knew I couldn't stay there. Finally, I made it off the bed and headed toward the door. Well, it was just a curtain. The rest of the BMT room was empty and dark. The rooms and the hallways were totally torn down to just the two by fours. The lights were construction lamps set up along yellow lines; plastic wallcovers were hanging all over as temporary walls. From there, I walked out of the BMT to the main floors—still no sign of people, everything dark and under construction. There were large groups of flying ants crawling on the floor. They looked pretty much like ants, with long slender wings. I could see rats scurrying along the bottoms of the walls. When I finally got to the main desk, there was a nurse there who I didn't recognize. She had an old classic nurse uniform on, and one of those little white hats. She reminded me of Nurse Ratched from *One Flew Over the Cuckoo's Nest*. There were a couple of patients and relatives of patients complaining about the situation, and all she kept saying was that the hospital was under construction and to go back to your rooms. When I got back to my room, it was in shambles—dust everywhere and no one to be found. I just stood there wondering what to do. As I stood, I looked out the window. Outside looked like a war zone. There were burnt buildings and smoke rising from them. No trees or grass just broken concrete and rubble. I guess being down at the sight of Ground Zero and seeing the destruction on 9/11 still lingered in my brain (yes, even 5 years later) as it does with all New Yorkers, or I suppose all Americans for that matter. As I looked, I thought maybe they finally got us again—9/11, part two.

To cheer myself up, I would watch plenty of comical movies and sitcoms. I had my regular schedule of shows to watch: *Seinfeld*, *King of the Hill*, and so on. My brother Steve brought me the whole collection of *The Little Rascals*. It helped a lot to laugh, and it just took my mind off of all the medical talk and mumbo jumbo.

On day 26 of my return to North Shore, I started developing a rash. By day 28, the rash was all over my body. My face was swollen and red. Maureen started calling me "Redman." Now I was the Redman. The rash wasn't exactly a bad thing. It was a sign that my body was adapting to the new marrow cells. It was something that the doctors *wanted* to see, but also didn't want to see it go too far out of hand. At the same time, I had been on high doses of steroids—very high—in order to adjust to the new blood. I found that the steroids made me very emotional. I still had my book and was almost finished with it. When I got to the part where Padre Pio died, I cried. My wife couldn't understand. She asked, "Why are you crying?" I said Padre Pio died. She thought it had to be something else and I said, "No that's it. He's been with me all this time, and now he's gone." I know it sounds weird, but it was just my belief.

Instead of getting all of my medications intravenously, they started tapering me off and I would receive pills and capsules. This is what I would rely on when I was home. I remember one night, when I was playing the war game on my computer and all you could hear were machine guns and bombs going off, one of the nurses came in—Eileen. I remember Eileen because she would always spend a lot of time with my mother and wife and talk about things that weren't related to the hospital all the time; that most likely was refreshing to them, rather than always talking about procedures. Anyway, she came into my room to give me my meds. Since I was so involved with the game, I asked her if it was OK if she came back later. She, in turn, replied "Sure, call me when you die." After a while, she realized what she had said and was kind of embarrassed.

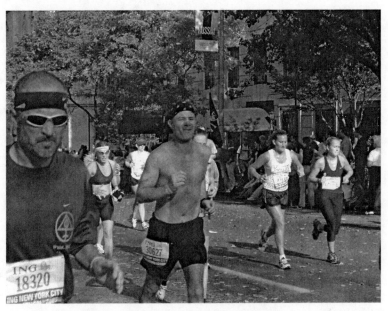

NYC marathon 2005

I didn't mind though. In fact, I thought it was funny. We both laughed about it afterwards.

My counts were beginning to rise and Dr. Bayer was very pleased with the outcome so far. My rash was almost gone (my face and neck were still red). Seemingly, it was nothing to worry about. Soon I would be discharged from the hospital and on my way home.

"Nothing can bring you peace but yourself"—Ralph Waldo Emerson

I would be home for Christmas. It wasn't much for me, compared to how I always felt during the Christmas season. I didn't care if I had seen anyone. My condition wasn't good. I was home, but there were rules to abide by. I was not allowed to leave the house, and the house had to be very clean; it was to be dusted every day, the bathroom cleaned with bleach, and the sheets changed at least 3 times a week. But not by me. I wasn't aloud to clean or dust. If I had to go out, I would wear a hospital mask and gloves. I wasn't allowed to eat food from the outside. Nothing. No restaurants, no food from the delis (rolls, Italian bread, cold cuts), no pizza or Chinese. I was not to be in crowds either. No church or the mall or any movie theaters. I really just had to stay secluded. Of course, I had to stay away from the sun. No swimming. I noticed my skin had changed; it was thinner, and there was no hair on my arms, legs, chest, or under my arms. My skin was lighter and smoother, and very tender. I was very vulnerable to cuts. On the tops of my hands, the skin was paper thin and very shiny. I would cut very easily and, with low platelets, take a long time to heal. Also, this is why I had to stay away from the sun. I was to live this way and be this way not for one month, not for six months, but for a complete year. My recovery wasn't finished. It wasn't just about getting new blood and returning to my normal life. There was still a risk. Mainly it was Host vs. Graf, and that means my body getting used to my new bone-marrow-making cells. It's like a total stranger coming to your house and living with you, and either you like him and you get along or you fight and argue and eventually throw him out. I would imagine my new blood mixing in my body like peanut butter and jelly, or a strawberry mix with milk. Just imagining everything in my body mixing together. As for medications, I had plenty progragh, celcept, Vfend, prednisone, mepron, valcyte, sleeping pills, pain killers, nausea pills and steroids. In total, 20 pills a day—10 in the morning and 10 at night.

I couldn't have pets in the house or plants, so Kika the cat had to go. Luckily my wife's sister Hilda agreed to take him.

As you can see, this was nothing like my first leave from the hospital, or my second. I was weak, very thin and didn't feel like doing anything.

During my transplant and afterwards, I still exercised as much as I could. While in my room at the hospital, I requested a stationary bike and used it almost every day. Also, I would jog in place for a good 15 to 20 minutes. Don't ask me how I did it, but I did. When I returned home, I bought a bike of my own and used it maybe once or twice a week. Still, I wasn't feeling good; I had very low energy.

When we bought the bike, it had to be assembled. Jhosber (my step son) and I decided to assemble it. It would have been a simple task for me in my normal condition. In this case, it was a different story. Every turn of a screw was a task in itself. Bending down and getting up again was so difficult. I felt like a 90-year-old man, having to take breaks every few minutes to catch my breath. I thought about how, a year ago, I was running marathons, and I wondered if I would ever be my old self again.

We did get it done. At least I accomplished something.

CHAPTER 15

Carolina Monti Saladino

Today is the December 29th 2006. A Friday. I am at the Monter Cancer Center. This is where I get my treatment, check my blood cultures and also see my doctor. I have been out of the hospital for 11 days so far. This is my third check up. Everything is going well. My blood counts are leveling off. Right now, what's happening is that the blood is changing from my bone marrow and generating into my blood stream. They are like baby blood cells and eventually they grow into adults. The whole process takes about a year. For me, right now, the hardest part is the medication. I have to take the pills, plus some liquid medication called Cyclosporine. Cyclosporine is one of the medications that helps mix my new blood into my body. The blood type of my donor is O. My blood type is A. Eventually I will no longer have my A blood. It will all be type O. Amazing, isn't it?

There is also a lab here. They take a blood sample every time I come here to see if I need blood or platelets. If I do, they give it to me. It's not bad; you sit in a small room with a recliner and a TV in it. Sometimes you can be here for hours. Today I'll be receiving my first dose of gamaglobin, so I'll be in the treatment room for about 3 to 4 hours.

In June of 1972, a 16-year-old named Don Monti died of Myeloblastic Leukemia. Within days of his death, his parents Joseph and Tita committed themselves to founding an organization in his memory, ultimately dedicated to finding a cure for cancer. While no cure has been found in the years since Don Monti's passing, much progress has been made.

Starting small, the Montis established steps that are still in place today and have helped thousands of patients directly, as well as an untold numbers who have benefited indirectly from the foundation's research and the expertise of their physicians. The first step was to establish the Don Monti Division of Oncology and Hematology at North Shore, where no such specialized service existed before. This division now treats more patients than any other in the region, and has offered even more treatment options through the Don Monti Bone Marrow Transplantation Unit. To further its scope and promise, Don Monti Cancer Centers have been opened in Huntington, Glen Cove, Forest Hills, Plainview, Franklin and Southside Hospitals.

I could imagine now how a mother must feel after losing her son to this devastating disease, and for that matter, a family. Four hours after the death of their son, Joseph, the father, took his wife in his arms and told her "we've got work to do." From there, the work began. Tita dedicated the rest of her life to working with the North Shore Hospital, creating the Don Monti Research Center. For nearly three decades, she came to her office 5 days a week, overseeing all the details—great and small—of the Don Monti Memorial Research Foundation. Mrs. Monti was born Tita Skandalis in Pelham, New York. The daughter of Greek immigrants, she began playing the piano as a child and performed in Carnegie Hall at the age of 11. Her singing voice matured and became dramatic soprano.

She gave up piano to coach voice at The Juilliard School of Music. There, she met and married Joseph Monti, a tenor. Mrs. Monti taught at the school for a decade and had three children: Caroline, Richard and Don. I unfortunately never met Tita, but did have the pleasure of meeting her daughter Carolina. Caroline, like her mother, has dedicated her life to curing cancer.

Today, the foundation raises more than $1 million annually—$35 million since its founding—and serves an ever-growing number of patients. Its commitment remains firm as the second and third generations of Montis, led by its president Carolina Monti Saladino, assume responsibility for its mission: research, education, fellowship, and patient care.

January 11th 2007…today is the 11th day of January, the day after my father's birthday. He's 74. Today was an honorable day for me. I went to my job. I've been out of the hospital for 3 weeks now and feeling good. I'm still not out of it yet, not by a long shot, but in my mind I believe I'm cured and getting stronger every day. I had spoken to my friend Will Biez a few days earlier, and he had told me that the drivers had raised a few dollars for me. I'm a bus driver for the NYC Transit Authority. Well, as I told you about these guys, they're friends, like family. I spoke to my union and told them I'd be back in June, so as of right now I'm still getting paid. The money has been getting a little low. By the way, I would strongly suggest to anyone: get yourself some accident insurance. I did, and it helped a lot. Hey, you never know.

Anyway, Willy had everyone gather in the crew room. The crew room looks something like a school cafeteria with the long stainless steel tables and benches and TV, and of course the vending machines. They installed a ping-pong table and a pool table for our sometimes long breaks in the day, and also to compensate for the stress of a busy driving day. Even the management was there (usually we stayed separate). I sat in a corner of the room, of course wearing my hospital mask and gloves, and just listened. He said that we are all family here and that one of our brothers had gotten very ill and it was time for us to help him. And they did. They raised over $3,000. I was honored. It felt good to see my friends and fellow bus drivers again.

As for my symptoms, I was doing as to be expected— very weak and still taking my 20 pills a day. One day, when I returned from the Monti Clinic, I received a phone call from Diane Kissinger informing me that I had inflammation of my liver. All the meds tend to do a number on your liver. So I had to get a liver biopsy. The biopsy was performed by a Dr. Benlevy. The biopsy was done right next door to the clinic. I thought the procedure was very interesting. What they do is they probe your body with a sonogram and get a picture of your liver. I watched on the screen and to me it looked pretty good; it looked like a pretty healthy liver, no spots, no fat...Anyway after they get a good picture, they take a long needle and stick it right into your stomach around the area just below your chest, and with the sonograph you can see it in there, probing for the liver. They stick the needle in the liver and abstract the chemical they need. Dr. Bayer wanted to make sure that I wasn't having problems with Graft vs. Host transferring in my body.

The next four to six months were crucial because everything had to mix correctly. I'd still imagine my peanut butter and jelly scenario. That's how I get through a lot of things in life; I imagine myself in the future. Alright, I'm in this situation now, but a year from now I'd see myself in my uniform and driving a bus. Think about this: say I'm running a marathon, let's say

NYC. I already know the course. I start out at the Verrazano Bridge running toward Brooklyn, then I picture myself entering downtown Brooklyn, and when I finally get there I'd do it again—next stop coming down Greenpoint Avenue and finally to the 59th Street Bridge. I always remember running over that bridge, mainly because the NYC marathon has so many spectators, but not on the bridge; that's the only spot where they don't allow spectators, so it's a quiet two-mile run over the bridge. I'd see myself running down the exit ramp onto First Avenue and the huge crowds cheering the runners on, then it's up First Avenue to Mile 20 where they have the Power Gel zone set up, and the bands. From there, again I'd see the future. I'd be in Harlem and the high school marching bands would be there, doing their part. Then finally down Fifth Avenue and into Central Park, and I can't wait to see that Mile 24 sign. Guess what? From there I see the finish line and myself running through with both hands held high. I did it—a complete marathon, 26.2 miles.

Actually, I kind of viewed my whole illness this way. Although it didn't work out exactly like I planned, in the long run it worked.

CHAPTER 16

Martina Keager

During my recovery years, 2006 through 2008, I had kept in touch with my new anonymous friend from Germany. Of course, as soon as I was released from the hospital, I sent a Christmas card. I knew very little about her—just that she was German and she was female. Other than that, it was all a mystery: her age, what she looked like (though in my mind I had a pretty good picture of what I thought she looked like), if she was married, if she had any children, and so on. We'd write inconspicuous letters to each other, trying to learn as much about each other as we were allowed to. When I received my first letter from her, I was very surprised, but also very pleased that she was interested in knowing how I was coming along.

MY FIRST LETTER FROM MY DONOR
To the person from this I hope so much that this will be totally health trough my bone marrow. Thank you very much for your card it was a great surprise and I am so much glad to hear from you. As it in the moment not possible to know your name and address come to know. I hope never the less further on this way have contact with you. Of course it is very difficult for me to correspond in English. However I have nice people those help me to read your letters. But if it is possible to write

in other languages (in //////) we can try it. How do you do and how long have you known about your illness? At the first moment I hoped and I wished that I could help you. After the inquiry about the bone marrow donates reach me. At once it was clear for me I will help equal what came up to me. I was 3 days in the hospital and I got all over well. But the very best moment was at I obtain your card and I knower it has been worthwhile and you'll be well. These 4 cards will be beyond the Christmas days have a place of honor. Not only I but my complete family. Wish you all goods above all that you can celebrate Christmas with your family and we wish your illness is past now.

May God now hold his guarded hands over you and may God give you only well and carefree days for months and many years. I hope that I hear again from you.

Even before my transplant, we had given cards to the Blood Donor Foundation and just hoped that the donor would receive our cards. Some donors don't expect to receive a card and also we weren't sure of a return letter. And as for us—Mom, Nubia and the family—we were very surprised and happy to hear from her. When I read the part where she had mentioned God, I believed that all our prayers were answered. My prayers, Mom's, Nubia's, Pop's, Aunt Bettie's, Rosalie's, Genie's, the Church's, Carolina's, Lilly's, The Koreans in Arizona, and the list goes on. We all thought as one.

I again wrote another letter to my donor to let her know how everything was working out:

Dear Donor,
To my friend from overseas, I was so happy to hear from you. I understand that you speak a different language. I know

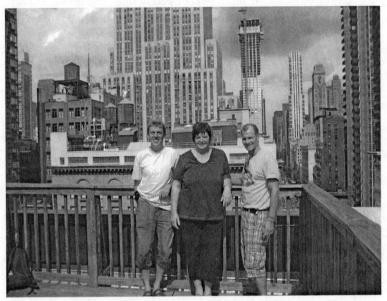

Andreas' Martina and me

English and my wife speaks Spanish, so I don't know if it will help, but I'll send this to you in Spanish also.

What can I say...I couldn't have done it without you. It was just you and one other person they found in the whole Donor Association. I don't know if you know that—only two people!

I'm doing fine. I received your donation on November 17ᵗʰ and stayed in the hospital until December 18ᵗʰ. I have been out of the hospital for 3 weeks now and feeling good. I am taking a lot of medication and have been weak, but it's to be expected. I see my doctor two, sometimes three, times a week to check my blood and my blood counts.

I will be 44 on February 17ᵗʰ so I'll see another birthday. As always, I thank God for everything and thank Him for sending you. I hope your children are fine and hope to hear from you soon.

God bless you and your family.

P.S. Feel free to write anytime!

Finally, after almost 3 years, in July of 2009 I got to learn the full identity of my bone marrow donor. Her name is Martina Keager. How did I learn? Well, one day I received a phone call from Diane Kissinger and she told me about how the bone marrow associations along with the Monter association were working on making arrangements for me to meet with my donor, Martina.

You see, every year North Shore Hospital holds a survivor dinner. And at this event, they choose a survivor to meet with their donor.

I remember the one year I had attended, a young man had met with his donor—a man that looked much older than the person that received his stem cells. Anyway, it seemed to have worked out fine. The night seemed to go by kind of quietly and nonchalantly. A few pictures were taken and I can't recollect if the survivor had made a speech or not. I like being invited to these meetings because I get to meet and talk with other survivors and hear their stories of survival. Also, I always wonder about how my fellow survivors that I shared time with in the hospital are doing, though rarely did I meet any. I asked the nurses about certain people who were fighting the leukemia monster alongside me, only to learn that they didn't do as well as I did. Jackie, the young girl of only 21 years, did not survive; she passed in 2010.

When Diane told me that they were trying to bring my donor here, all the way from Germany, I had my doubts. As the days passed, we learned more about the whole meeting. But nothing was for sure. Diane asked me if I had stayed in touch with my donor and when was the last time I had heard from her. Well, the only way we stayed in touch was by writing anonymous letters to each other. Mom had also written numerous letters to her but had gotten nothing in return for months. I told Diane the situation. The next time I returned to the clinic, Diane gave me a consent form permitting us to learn each other's names, as well as where we lived. I filled out the form, but did not hear from Martina for a few months. And even though we did not hear from her, the hospital was still working on our meeting.

In July, I received a letter from my donor with a book of the country she lived in as well as some pictures. This is the letter:

My name is Martina Keager. I hope you still know me. I am very glad to get your email address and it is now possible to contact you. Exactly on my birthday I have received your name and your address. This was a very nice present for me. I know now that you and your family does well. I would like to introduce you to my family; my husband called Andreas—he is 41 years old. We have two sons Stefan and Tobias, Tobias is 11 and Stefan is 9. We live together in Bavaria on the border of Germany, in a small village named Runding. It is near the border of the Czech Rep. I would like to send you in the next days a book about my country and a few pictures of myself. Of course I will be very happy if I heard from you and your family too. I had get a letter from your mother in Germany—was she living in Germany for 45 years? Do you have a person who can speak and write in German? Because my English is not very good. Because our visit in Sept—we will check this term and will give you an information. I want to visit you with my husband.

Mom had written a few letters to Martina using a friend to translate the letter into the language. Well, she didn't quite get it right, becuase actually she was in Germany for just 4 or 5 days. We all got a kick out of this. I joked with Mom, "You mean you lived in Germany and you still didn't know the language?"

I often would browse through the book that Martina had sent me and look at the pictures of her and her family. How different it seemed compared to the big city—the huge mountains of the Alps, the tremendous waterfalls and lakes, the vast fields with just a tiny house in the middle of it, and how they must have had to travel tens of miles just to buy bread and milk. I thought about just how far it must have been to travel to the hospital. For me, it was a 15-minute ride. So if I were to receive a letter, it wasn't a big deal. The hospital ride for Martina to receive it must have been a full day's journey.

As the weeks went by and I had made my doctor's visits, I found it was true: she would be here for the survivor's dinner and I was to be the main focus of the night.

The date was September 23rd. Now I was counting the days. My next doctor's visit was on the September 17th. Now whenever I went to the Clinic it was always with my head held high and full of smiles. I thought of the past, my times in the

treatment room being pumped with Gamaglobin or receiving
blood or platelets or some other type of medication and having
to sit there for hours. Now I felt as though I was visiting all my
friends, like Fran, one of the receptionists who had jet black
hair, would always greet me with a smile, even when I was
at my worst. She would always ask me about my motorcycle
and if I did any riding lately. She likes motorcycles. And the
nurses' aides in the examining room where they would take
my vitals—one woman named Farah, who was originally from
Iran, would tell me about their crazy President. She had this
high-pitched laugh where everyone in the room would hear
us laugh together. And then of course Dr. Bayer and Diane.
I remember sitting in the waiting room and Diane always
trying to find me. She would usually find me by one of the
windows, either lying down on the bench (because back then
I was always tired and weak and she'd always make sure I
had the mask and gloves on right) or just leaning against the
window, holding myself up. Well, this day was different. I did
my usual thing: got my blood checked, said hello to everyone
and sat down in my usual seat. Before I knew it, I was in the
exam room with Dr. Bayer and Diane. We didn't really talk
about me. It was mostly about Martina and the big party, what
time she would arrive, where she would stay, and how long. I
have to say: they seemed very excited about the whole ordeal.
My doctor told me that she was going to say a speech and a
little something about me. I told her about my book and how I
had kept a journal since day one of my diagnosis. She said that
she would like to read a bit of it and use it in her speech. She
also told me that it would be nice if I said a little something. I
didn't want to. I'm really not that type of guy who likes to give
speeches. But deep down, I thought everyone should know
how I felt. Oh, by the way, my counts were good. I went home,

got my journal and my book and pictures from Martina, and delivered it to Dr. Bayer.

In the next few days, while I was working, I received a call from my local news station in Queens—I think it was Channel 12. The woman asked me all kinds of questions. How did I know I had leukemia? How long was my stay in the hospital? And did I have contact with my donor? I thought, "wow, I might be in the Queens newspaper."

I decided to take a few days off from work (I had been at work almost a full year now) and take my donor out on the town. Also, I thought about writing my speech and finally got the words I wanted to say.

September 23rd had arrived. The day felt like any other. It was a beautiful day in September. The temperature was in the 70s with clear skies.

I thought back a few years earlier, to 2007, when I was to attend my first survival dinner. That was 10 months after my BMT and I really didn't feel up to it. Still, I dressed in my best suit and tie and waited for my wife to get home from work. The weather was cold, wet and storming; I had never seen it as bad as it was that night. The water was almost up to the first step of the front entrance to my house. We made a commitment, so we decided to make the journey to the outskirts of Long Island. Well, with the rain came the flooding and the mad traffic. We tried short cuts and detours until we eventually got lost. I was never good at navigating in Long Island anyway. I'm originally a Bronx boy. Finally, after two hours of driving, we decided to call it quits and make our way back home. I didn't want to make the night a total failure for me and Nubia, so I thought if Dr. Bayer allowed me to eat at the dinner (remember, I was not allowed to eat on the outside for one full year) I guessed she wouldn't mind if I ate somewhere else. We picked up the kids, Jhosber and Jhoanna, and found a nice restaurant on Northern Boulevard, next to our home in Queens. For starters I had pizza, and topped it off with my favorite dish, chicken cutlet parmesan, of course. And I had dessert: a piece of cake and cappuccino.

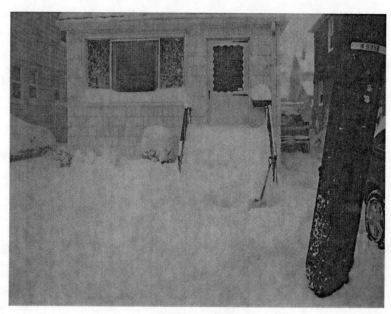

winter of 2006

CHAPTER 17

Back to the Future: 2009

Health-wise, I felt so different. I was stronger and more energetic. I was running, almost at my normal pace. I also joined the Parks Department Health Club and was swimming. My weight wasn't up to par though. I was at 163. Still, I felt good.

The newswoman who had called me a few times asked me if we could get to the dinner a little early so she could interview us beforehand. I had gotten a new suit (which we had picked up in Philadelphia after seeing an Elton John and Billy Joel concert at Citizens Bank Park). And my wife was in a nice looking dress. We left the house at 4:30, stopped to get flowers for Martina, and got there at about 5:10. The place was a very elegant manor in Long Island called The Crest Hallow Country Club. It had big chandeliers and a grand piano in the lobby, with granite tiles on the floor and in the bathrooms. It's owned by the Monti Family. We drove up the driveway to the main entrance, and went in. It was like lights, camera, action. As soon as Nubia and I entered, the flash bulbs went off and the cameras were rolling. The news lady directed us straight to a sort of waiting room where there was cold water and soda. The media had set it up. They didn't want us to see each other beforehand; I guess they really wanted the element of surprise. We waited two to three minutes until a tall, dark-skinned lady, who looked to be in her late forties, entered the room. Her name was Joy Brown and she was a columnist for New York *Newsday*. Diane was at her side and said, "This is Joy Brown from NY *Newsday* and she'd like to ask you a few questions." They were the usual—how are you feeling at the moment, how long did you keep in touch, and how long have you been in remission? Well, Diane and my wife pretty much helped me out with the questions, considering they knew my story as well as I did.

Shortly after that, we were escorted into what looked like the lounge of the country club. There were couches and chairs set up here and there, with those big needle-leafed fern plants all over. They had closed the two large entrance doors behind me. Now the reporters were at it again with the routine questions, but also setting the stage for when Martina would enter and figuring which angle would be best to shoot. I overheard one of the reporters saying that she was here. In a few minutes, she entered the room and the flash bulbs went off. She must have felt like a real celebrity. Martina was a tall woman, about my height—5'9"—and very healthy looking. She had dark brown hair like mine, and brown eyes like mine. Her face was as I had pictured it: a round, high-cheeked German face.

I turned to her, gave her a bouquet of flowers, and thanked her for all she had done for me. Now we were standing side-by-side with the news media surrounding us, asking questions back and forth. By this time, I felt myself start rambling, saying how emotional I was and how this whole scenario from my diagnosis onwards had felt like a dream with a happy ending.

As dinnertime rolled around, I met and spoke to some of my old nurses and a few patients that were in the hospital at the same time I was. The room was full of survivors and their families. All in all, I would say it was a good 300 people eating and just talking about life. I would think most of them were probably talking about their own life stories. We ate appetizers like fruits, cheeses and diced cold cuts. At dinner, it was a choice between chicken and fish. I had the fish.

In time, a couple of survivors told their stories. I remember one of them who was there at the same time I was. I think his name was Bill. He was a tall, older man, maybe in his sixties. We never actually spoke, though I had seen him in the Monter Center. Then, a dark-haired woman spoke. She was diagnosed with her illness in 2003. They all told their stories about life and how they valued each day. Then came Dr. Ruthie Lu Bayer. As always, she thanked her staff and the other doctors. She then asked them to come up front, so they could be recognized. Then everyone applauded. When the crowd stopped clapping, she told my story and how I felt about my mother, my daughters and my best friend, Nubia. She talked about my life as a bus driver, as a father, and as a runner.

The way she told it was really heartfelt. I mean, the news interviews, waiting to meet Martina, and finally meeting her didn't hit me as hard as Dr. Bayer did when she told my story. I felt it in my heart. She talked about Martina and how difficult it was for her to get to the hospital. When she finished, she asked us to stand. Everyone applauded. Then we both walked up to the front of the room. I held her by the hand. Ruthie Lu asked me if I would like to say a few words. I had written my speech, had practiced it a few times, and if I didn't say it then, I knew I would regret it for a long time.

MY SPEECH

Dear friends, family and especially survivors, today has to go down as one of the most unforgettable days of my life. Three years ago, in June 2006, I was diagnosed with AML and was just devastated about the news. I couldn't believe it. I thought, how could this be? I always ate right, exercised daily, and even ran marathons, so I thought there must be some mistake. But it was true. True enough to go through chemotherapy and finally a bone marrow transplant. None of it was easy, as we all know in this room. We searched nationwide for a donor. None were found—not in New York, not California, none in the U.S. But the Bone Marrow Association, my doctor Dr. Bayer, and of course Diane didn't give up on me. They went international and in October 2006 I found a donor. My prayers were answered. The person they had found was from Europe, a person who didn't know me. We didn't speak the same language. But the person was caring enough to give. We kept in touch with each other since the transplant, not knowing each other's name or age or exactly where we were from. Finally, last July, we found out each other's name and the place we lived.

Her name is Martina Keager—yes, a female—and she is from Germany. This explains my craving for knockwurst and sauerkraut. Today is the day we finally met and there is at least one word I can say to her in German: danke schoen, which means thank you.

My story isn't quite over yet. You see, I vowed that if I ever got better I would run another marathon. So, in January 2010, I am going to do it. Not for myself, but for the people who are still suffering from this disease and hoping for a cure.

The rest of the night we danced.

A few notes about my unforgettable night. We made the *New York Daily News* and also *Newsday*. Not to mention Channels 11, 12, 4 and 5, plus 1010 WINS news radio. But the thing that I always will remember, and found the most extraordinary, is that September 23rd is the feast day of St. Padre Pio. I didn't realize it until that night. Nubia got a phone call from my step-daughter Jhoanna from school saying that she was attending the mass for St. Padre Pio at her school.

Martina had full days in our city of New York. I wanted to make the best of it for her, so after the party I said to

Martina and her husband Andreas, "Be prepared for a long day tomorrow. Nubia and I will pick you up at 9am." They were staying at a quaint motel in Great Neck, Long Island. It was close to the Long Island Rail Road, so it was easy access to the city.

The next day, 9am came and we were at the door of the motel. Martina and Andreas were already waiting in the lobby. From there, we parked and strolled to the train station. As we were buying tickets, we noticed *New York Newsday* had our story. I bought 3 copies and Martina did the same. The newspaper man looked at us kind of strangely. I just said, "It's a good newspaper." All four of us laughed. We hopped on the train and in about 25 minutes we were at Penn Station—34th Street and Seventh Avenue—also the address of Madison Square Garden. And also the last stop of the Q32 bus. Off the train we went and up the stairs to the many stores underground. Starbucks, TGI Fridays, pizzerias, sandwich shops, even Duane Reade. Once outside, we crossed Seventh Avenue with the other hundreds of people heading to work. I couldn't help thinking of how our guests must have felt at this moment, coming from a small town in Germany. As we got to the other side where all the buses were parked, some of my colleagues noticed us as we were walking and said hello. They also said that they had seen us on the news last night.

We walked down 32nd Street toward Nubia's office, as she had to work that day. We left her at the door to her office building on the corner of 31st and Fifth Avenue. I kissed her goodbye and told her that we would be back for lunch. We walked on and Martina browsed through some of the small souvenir shops. The first stop was the mall on 34th and Sixth Avenue. Andreas bought American jeans, which he said cost a fortune in Germany, and sneakers for his sons (Yankee sneakers). From there, we hit the Empire State Building. Did you know that you have to take three elevators to get to the top? Andreas had his camera and was taking pictures at every stop. By the way, if you're wondering how we communicated with each other, Andreas' English was very good. He told me that he had learned in high school, but after that he never really spoke it much. I was surprised that he knew so much.

When we finally got to the top of the great building (which I hadn't been to since I was a boy), the view was, of course, spectacular. All you could see, from every point of view, were rows and rows of skyscrapers, and on the outskirts were the two rivers on each side—the Hudson and the East River. I acted as if I were their tour guide, pointing out the park (Central Park) and all the famous rivers and buildings. After that, it was back to Nubia for lunch. Nubia works for an advertising agency and the building is in a pretty cool spot on Fifth Avenue. There's a little roof-deck at the top, with a great view up Fifth Avenue. Of course we took pictures. We went for lunch on 32nd Street, which is known as Korea-town, so of course we had Korean food. I had pork ribs and rice. Nubia knew of some special Korean plates—basically it was small, round bowls with spicy foods and vegetables. Different, but good.

We spent an hour with Nubia, and then it was back on the tour of the town. We walked back down toward Penn Station where the buses were parked and I searched for someone I knew. I wanted to take them to Central Park. We got lucky and found a fellow Casey Stengel Bus Depot driver who actually was going out of service and offered us a ride to the park. We had the whole bus to our selves. As we rode up Madison Avenue to the park, again I thought about how Martina must have felt, riding a city bus on our own, in the middle of Manhattan. We were dropped off at 57th and Madison. We walked through Central Park and ended up at the Central Park Zoo. We didn't actually go in, but from the path we could see some polar bears swimming, and we saw the clock with the zoo animals on it, where every half hour the animals spin and dance slowly to the music. We climbed a hill in the park and just sat a while and drank soda.

Our day wasn't over yet. Next was the Statue of Liberty. We grabbed another friendly bus driver who took us back to 34th Street, and from there we caught the M7 bus to Battery Park. As we got on the bus, a couple of passengers recognized us from TV and offered me good luck and health in my life. We passed Ground Zero, and still every time I pass there I think of that day that destroyed the lives of more than you would think.

Finally, we made it to Battery Park. I took the cheap way out. My finances weren't that great at the time (and still aren't), so instead of taking the ferry to the island we hopped on the Staten Island Ferry. The ferry is free (don't tell anyone) and it goes right past the statue. Again, Andreas had his camera out. We returned to 32nd Street one more time, picked up Nubia—now it was close to 5:30—and before getting back on the LIRR we stopped at TGI Fridays and had a few beers and talked about the day. It was a good day.

On day two, we stayed in Queens. This time we went to Flushing Meadow Park, where they had the World's Fair. We saw the sphere and also the towers, which, if you remember, were in the movie *Men in Black*. We walked to the lake, and saw the tennis courts where the U.S. Open takes place. Of course, Andreas was there with his camera. We took a break at the golf course and then went to my house for lunch. We barbecued in the back yard—hot dogs, hamburgers and fries. Just the three of us.

I believe my family and I showed our new friends from Germany a fantastic and memorable time in our great city. We ate dinner in Little Italy the last night, and stood in the middle of Times Square. What a view, and what a time to remember.

CHAPTER 18

The Marathon

Early in September 2009, while riding my usual bus route, I noticed an ad on one of the panels above the passenger seats. It was an ad for Team in Training. The ad was purple, with a woman running on the side. Straight away it caught my attention. Running was a suggestion for participating in an endurance competition. Either a triathlon—swimming, biking and running—or a biking century, which is 100 miles. Or you could run a full or a half marathon. Well, here's the kicker: it was all to raise money for the Leukemia Society. I thought about Jen and how she had run a marathon in honor of me. Now it was my turn to help. I had been working a little over 6 months at the time and really thought I was ready. So, without any hesitation, I made the phone call. I made arrangements for the winter season training. In all, I had to raise $3,800 dollars for charity. If everything went well, I would be running the Miami Marathon.

The first meeting was held in a library in Astoria, Queens. To me, it seemed kind of odd, only because most of the 20 to 30 people there, if not all of them, had never really even run a mile before. Then I figured it out. They just wanted to help, but didn't know how. Like me, they had seen firsthand what this disease can do to a person. They all had their own stories of loved ones who suffered one way or another from cancer—aunts, uncles, mothers, fathers, sisters, brothers, and so on. I figured that after seeing the hospital beds and the people suffering in them with cancer and getting huge doses of chemo that makes them even worse for a while, after seeing all that they could suffer the pain of running a marathon to help.

After we committed ourselves, October was the first big meeting. It was in Manhattan, and I'd say over 100 people showed. Still, most were there in honor of a special person in their life and of course they asked the question "are there any survivors here" and about 10 of us stood up and were asked to come to the front. We all had our stories. Most had it when they were very young, and I remember there was one young boy there with his mother—he must have been about 5 or 6. He had been dealing with his cancer for a few years already and his mother said, "He has his good days and bad," with a lump in her throat. We all spoke and told our stories of survival and why we were participating. Of course, mine was that in 2006 I was diagnosed with AML and vowed that if I ever got better I'd run another marathon. Well, from there, the rest was all running, and of course meeting new people and friends. As you know, I had been running for a while, but now it meant something.

I set up a facebook page to tell my story and start my fundraising. Nubia and I made flyers to put up in the bus depot, explaining how I was going to run to raise money for the Leukemia Society. Mom helped out too, even though she wasn't too thrilled about me running so early into my recovery. She went to her church and the Scottish Country Dancing Society where she dances, and the fundraising began. As for the running (which I thought of as the easy part compared to the fundraising), I did my own thing—except for Saturdays when I would meet with Team in Training. Before every run, we would get inspiration from someone there who had a friend or family member that was affected by leukemia. Then we ran. Mostly we ran in Central Park. It was great running that course—first, because I was running it again and second, I reminisced about the many times I would run the races here.

The advanced runners started out at one lap around the park, which added up to 6 miles. From there, we would add a mile every week. Back in my own running grounds in Queens, weekdays it was Flushing Meadows Park—I would do 7 to 10 miles—and on the weekends I'd add a few more, mainly at Alley Pond Park, which was very hilly. As for T.N.T we added a mile or two every time we met. I'd take the 7 train every Saturday morning and we met at the Central Park Band Shell at 8am. I had my own running group that I would run with; we were the top runners on the team. There was Jeremy, our mentor, a tall young guy in his 30s who had worked with T.N.T for a while. He not only ran marathons, he also ran triathlons. Then there was another Anthony; this was his first marathon. He was a tall, thin kid with dark hair and glasses. I'd also say he was in his late 20s or 30s. And there was Andrew, another young man. He was a fair-skinned guy with light blonde hair who was very quiet. And of course there was Pete. He was another young guy, compared to me. I was the old guy in the group. Pete was the guy everyone got along with and everyone knew. In total, there were about 80 of us.

Pete was the first guy I met with T.N.T. My first run in the park was with him and a girl named Helena. While we ran, we would talk to each other to take our minds off the run and pass the time. I don't like to bring it up, but I guess it ends up happening; I told my story of my fight against cancer.

I had told them about Martina and how we finally met each other for the first time, after 3 years of my ordeal, just a few weeks ago. When I told them, Pete realized who I was and said he remembered seeing us on the news. Helena also thought it was a great story. She suggested that I say something to the other runners. I told her I would, but I never did. I felt I would be wearing what had happened to me as a medal, and I really didn't want that. I wanted to be like everyone else there. Now I was running for someone else. I was running for all the patients at North Shore who I met, in honor of the ones that were still with us and in memory of the ones who had passed.

I ran. My runs in Central Park were getting longer and longer in preparation for the marathon. The main thing about running a marathon is the training. Before the big race, you must get your miles in. We ran inside and outside the park (literally). One of the more significant runs that I remember was an 18-mile long distance run. It was a very cold winter morning, as I recollect, in the low 30s. It was the end of November. The run started out at the Central Park Band Shell at our usual time, 8:30. We took a trail that led outside of the park and made a left down 79th Street to the West Side Highway. The West Side Highway has a running path especially made for runners, bikers and walkers. We were in a group of about 7. It was my usual group: Jeremy, Anthony, Andrew, Pete, and a few others. Our run went from Central Park all the way to the Brooklyn Bridge. And of course we couldn't stop there; we had to go over it. As we got to the other side, the time was close to 10am. At the end of the bridge was a small diner. Even though the temperature was in the 30s, when you're running that far you still need to drink plenty of liquids, so when we got to the other side I thought it was a good time to use the bathroom. So, I went into the diner and this little diner was packed with patrons having their weekend brunch. I thought, look at me, running 18 miles in 30-degree weather in the middle of the winter, while most people in the city are just waking up and enjoying their weekend. Then I remembered why I was doing it. Hey, I was there for six months straight in the hospital, with four horrendously strong doses of chemo and all the side effects that go along with it—the fevers, the headaches, pneumonia, diarrhea and constipation, the vomiting and nausea. Yes, I knew why. And also my running partners knew. They weren't there to run 26 miles. They were there because they had a cause they wanted to help in any way they could. And we did.

CHAPTER 19

Train, Endure, Achieve, Matter!

Train, Endure, Achieve, Matter! This was our Anthem. We wanted to make a difference. We all, in our hearts, were fighting cancer. On January 9th 2010, about 30 of us showed up at LaGuardia Airport in New York for a 3-day trip to Miami to run the Miami Marathon. I was ready. I had gotten my miles in, and again I was in great shape. I brought some motorcycle magazines for the plane, and of course I had my friends. It's less than a 2-hour flight from NY to Florida. When we arrived, we were consumed by the total difference in the weather. We went from training in 20 to 30-degree weather to 70 to 80 degrees and humid in Florida. Straight away I knew it was going to be a tough one.

We hopped on the bus and arrived at our hotel. It was a really extravagant hotel—a 300 dollar a night hotel. How did I know? Well, I asked to stay an extra night, and that didn't work out too well. It had grand pianos in the lobby and waterfalls—a little too pricey for my wallet. What was good about it was that the beginning and the end of the marathon was right down the street from the hotel. My room was on the tenth floor, and I shared it with another runner who I hadn't met before. He was a really tall guy—I'd say about 6'6"— with curly brown hair. He was a lot younger than I was, maybe in his late 20s. His name was also Anthony. We talked a bit, but mostly I stayed with Jeremy, his girlfriend Kristin, and my other running partners. That Friday night, we walked the little walkway that was next to the hotel, which had restaurants, bars and gift shops. One good thing about running a marathon is that you have to eat a lot of carbs before the race; running that many miles, you burn it all. So we hit the Italian restaurants the first night. I think I ate a whole pie. By the way, no alcohol, though it would have been nice to have had a few beers.

Saturday it was off to the convention center, which was in South Beach, Miami. We walked by the beach, where they have all the tables for dining on the sidewalk. Breakfast was a spinach omelette, potatoes, toast some fruit, and I threw in some pancakes. From there, we walked to the center to pick up our gear for the race—a race number, a tag for the shoe, and a shirt. They had all kinds of vendors there for all your running needs, from running shoes to rain gear. They had those bracelets that are supposed to improve your balance. There were people speaking and they also had a video of the whole course. That night was the pasta party—all-you-can-eat spaghetti. There were speeches and they spoke about how much the Leukemia Society contributed to fighting the disease.

Before calling it a night, we had one last meeting with our NY team, pretty much just about what to prepare for. One thing the team physical therapist had told us was to make sure to drink a lot of fluids, especially due to the weather, and also to carb up before the race. Usually you'd have a bagel or something of that nature. Wake up was at 4:30am, so after that it was up to my room for a good night's sleep. Of course, before a big race, it's not that easy. I slept and I also dreamt. What did I dream of? What else. The marathon. I dreamt I had

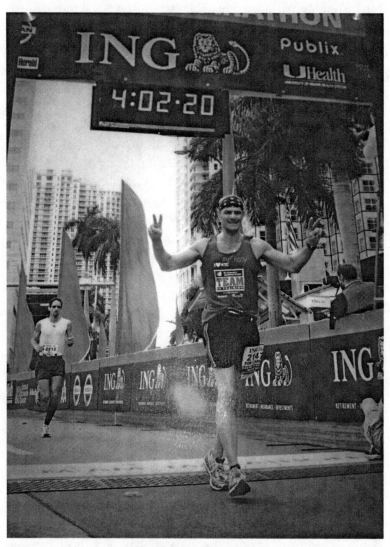

Miami Marathon 2010

missed the wakeup call and when I woke up the time was close to 9:00. I remember running to the window, looking out and seeing a sea of purple shirts running by (the Team in Training color is purple). I quickly changed into my shorts, purple T-shirt and running shoes, and ran for the elevator. It seemed as if the elevator wasn't working. I waited and waited and kept hitting the down button, but it was to no avail; the elevator did not come. Time for the stairs. I ran down the stairs, skipping two at a time, and sometimes I'd jump a whole flight. I went flight to flight, it seemed I must have gone at least 20 flights down, but never found the lobby. I turned and decided to go back up, thinking I must have passed it. This time, going up, I was skipping two to three steps at a time, trying to find the lobby. I couldn't find it. I decided to exit the stairwell and try the elevator again, and it just so happened that the floor I had gotten off on was the main floor. I wasted no time and ran to the starting gate, which was about half a mile away from the hotel. When I finally arrived, the place was empty—nothing there but empty Poland Spring bottles on the ground, along with some used Power Gel packets and the yellow tape on the sides of the road that creates the lanes. I noticed a gentleman with long black hair and round-rim sunglasses who reminded me of John Lennon, sitting where the starting gate was with the time clock over it. The clock read 3 hours 59 minutes. He was sitting by the empty bleachers. I approached him and asked him if I could still run the race. The race clock was approaching its fourth hour. He said, "You can, but it won't count. You're too bloody late. If I were you, I'd go back home." I stood there for a minute or two thinking how could I have missed it, after all my training, this was my race, and then walked back to the hotel.

Just then, there was a knock at the door. It was 4:30am, January 31st 2010. Race day!

It was a humid, hot morning, close to 70 degrees. The race was to begin at 6:30am sharp. Due to the weather, they started extra early. I had taken note of what the physical therapist of the team had told us. I had my Gatorade in hand. As usual, I'd drink a 32-ounce fruit punch. But also, for a change, I figured I'd get my carbs in; the night before I had ordered room service: two toasted bagels with cream cheese. Before every marathon, you try and figure out ways to improve from your last run. Some people are superstitious and do certain things before the race—eat the same meals, drink a coffee and a donut, go to mass the day before, and so on. 26 miles is a long journey.

We all met in the lobby of the hotel at 5am, took pictures with the team, and then it was off to the starting gate. It was still dark out at this time of year. I remember walking with Anthony and Andrew, the quiet guy, to the start. It was very dark and all you saw were small groups of people here and there, walking and talking and laughing to themselves. Then some on their own, walking, or on the side, stretching. Everyone was in their own strange mood—excited, scared, nervous, and probably thinking "what the hell am I doing here?" Me, I was ready to run. 2006 was my last marathon. That was 4 years ago.

We were set up in corals according to our mile time. Anthony, Andrew and I were set in the same coral at the 8 minute mile mark. Jeremy was in the sevens; he was competing for a chance to enter the Boston Marathon. I think he had to run a 3:20 race.

In all, there were about 10,000 of us. There were speeches from some recent marathoners for inspiration, then the Mayor of Miami. I remember beach balls being thrown around to try and kill our anticipation for the race, as we were all waiting for the National Anthem to be sung and then the loud horn for the start.

The three of us had our adrenaline flowing through us, so Anthony and Andrew took off (it was their first marathon). I said, "Hey guys, slow it down, we got a long way to go." The race was basically a great 26-mile figure 8. We started out at the city of Miami and then went south towards South Beach, which was close to 7 miles. Still, we were running in the dark. Anthony and Andrew kept bursting ahead and I eventually lost them in the crowds of runners.

It's funny; even though you're running, you still get to meet and talk with other people along the way. There was a young woman who was running next to me and noticed my purple Team in Training shirt, on the back of which I had hand-written FOR CARLA. I know, right now you're thinking to yourself, who's Carla? One of my colleagues at the bus depot, Frank Tufunkjien, came to visit me while I was in the hospital— actually when I was receiving my transplant—and told me that his wife also had it. Yes, AML. This was in 2006. Carla had gotten a stem cell transplant using her own stem cells (antilogous) but the cancer slowly returned. What a feeling that must be...to go through the chemo and the transplant, only to have this unforgiveable disease return. After that, in 2008, I visited her in the hospital and reassured her that with a transplant from a donor (allergenic) she would survive. She was very happy to see me and hear my words of support. She did receive a BMT from her brother, who was a match, and I hear she is doing well. I still visit cancer patients and talk on the phone with them on occasion. I dedicated my marathon to Carla. I told the woman the story, not mentioning that I was also a cancer patient. We ran and talked for a while, but her stride was a little too slow for me, so I left her behind and searched for two other purple shirts.

At the time, we were running along a four-lane highway, so it was wide and full of runners. I noticed my companions to my left, not much farther away from me, and caught up. We ran as a threesome to South Beach. By then, the sun was rising and the heat and humidity were setting in. There were morning sprinklers for the grass, so I thought it was a good idea to run through them and cool off. I knew I had to stay cool for the long haul. Also, I wore a bandana to stop the sweat from getting in my eyes, and I poured water on my head to keep cool. The South Beach strip was very quiet. I thought there would have been more people on the sidewalks, cheering the runners on. Instead, it was eerily quiet. We were running by the ocean, which was nice. Also, it was the strip where the nightclubs were located. It seemed like the people that were on the street were just getting out of the clubs and were wondering what the heck was going on. I greeted them with a "Good Morning" and kept running. We were closing at mile 7 when I started feeling nauseous and realized it was the two cream cheese bagels I had eaten earlier, and thought maybe that wasn't the brightest thing to do. By mile 10, I was really feeling it. Also, at mile 10, we started seeing runners on the side of the road, passing out because of the heat or some other type of problem. We had a good stride going at this point, calculating that we were running at a 8 to 81/2 minute mile. So I wasn't stopping for a little stomach ache. As we got to mile 13, it was now more than the stomach that was bothering me. Now it was the heat. Still, we were running in a parallel line— three purple shirts in a row. At this point, we were on our way back to the starting gate. For the half marathoners, their day was complete. For us, it was another hot long 13 miles more.

We would be running out to Coconut Grove, on the outskirts of Miami. As we approached the finish line for the half, the crowds were big and all cheering us on, especially T.N.T. That gave me a little push to keep going. As we ran farther west, the crowds thinned out again until we were running down an empty highway. The nausea was still there, so I slowed down my pace as my companions ran on. At this point, the runners were sparse and I was absolutely on my own. Then another problem set in: as I had been pouring water on my head and body, and also running through the lawn sprinklers, I got my socks and shoes wet, so I was running in wet, soggy shoes. Naturally, my feet became very sore. But this was race day. Now, like everything else, I had to deal with it (winners never quit).

Coconut Grove was mostly residential, with the Floridian houses by the water and the palm trees in the front. You couldn't ask for better scenery. Most of the people who owned the houses were out in front with their kids and family, cheering for us to finish and handing out slices of oranges or bananas and cold bottles of water, saying, "Come on, you can do it—only 10 miles to go!" And I'd think to myself, *only*.

Believe it or not, I was still at a pretty good pace. I caught up with Anthony and asked him how he was doing. Like me, he was feeling the heat, and stopped and walked a while. We ran for the next mile, but he had a better stride and ran ahead. I guess we were on the main street of Coconut Grove. It was kind of a circular section, or I guess it was how the course was laid out, but we ended up running by the outdoor restaurants with people out eating, having a few cold drinks for Sunday brunch and gazing at the runners passing by. From there, it was back to the city of Miami and the finish line. My energy level was really running low at this point. Well, this wouldn't be the first time I felt this way. This was marathon number five, and for me they are never a cake walk.

It was a long, straight away strip to mile 20. I ended up falling in with a group of young runners in their 20s. They had a sign held up that read "330" meaning that that was the time in which they wanted to finish their run. They had a running coach with them. An older Spanish man with long grey hair and a dark tan was keeping the pace and chanting to them, "We are the best, 330 is the best, we will do it, let's go 330." I hung with them to mile 20. Then slacked off. The last six miles was two miles out onto what seemed like a long peninsula with a highway going out to who knows where, and you could see the runners coming back on the other side of the highway. I was making pretty good time. At this point, I was at 2:48 with just six miles to go. But this, as they say, is where you hit the wall. And I did. With my feet and my energy level down to, I'd say, less than half, I had to stop and walk. All the Power Gels and Gatorade couldn't help me now. All that was left was determination to finish. The rest of the way was a walk and run. I made it back to the end of the peninsula and there was then just two miles left to the finish. I made it to the 25 mile marker and remember catching up to an older Spanish man with glasses. I spoke to him, saying "This is it—the last mile." He said, "Yes and it's the hardest one." I responded, "Not for me."

I did it. I sprinted past him and didn't stop. I remember running over a long, steel, grated bridge and rounding a few streets on my way to the finish, with the crowds cheering at full volume. The last mile seemed never-ending. Then I saw it: the finish line. I kept my steady stride to the finish, holding my hands high over my head, making my "V for victory" sign, and my head up. What a feeling. I did it. 26.2 miles. Dr. Savanna was right. He and the hospital got me back running again.

SOME THINGS ABOUT THE RACE:
I finished at a time of 3 hours, 59 minutes, 58 seconds.
Anthony and Andrew both finished ahead of me.
Jeremy never finished because of heat exhaustion at mile 13.
Overall, out of the 80 New York runners, I came in third place.
Out of 2,871 runners, I placed 724.

There are many reasons why I wrote this book. My main reason was to make people aware of the importance of bone marrow transplants. In my opinion without one most leukemia patients will not survive. A story I heard recently is the type of thing you hear time and time again. This time it was about a girl who needed a liver transplant and the insurance company didn't finance it in time, so she eventually died. Later on, I found out that the girl also had leukemia. Well, in time, without the transplant, the monster ate away at the liver until it wasn't good any more. I believe if she had found a donor soon enough, she would not have needed the liver transplant. It's so easy to be a donor and you're a true lifesaver. During my illness, my wife, as I wrote in the book, coordinated a bone marrow drive and now, a year later, one of the people who donated was called by the Leukemia Society and was a match. She got the call.

I feel happy because, through my illness, someone might be saved. I'm hoping that, since I can never do it myself, maybe I can get other people to realize the great importance of donating.

I also wrote this book as a guide for other people who have, unfortunately, contracted this deadly blood disease—to help them see that it's not over and let them know, through my experience, what will happen during the way, what to do, and what not to do.

Additionally it's in written to honor the memory of my friends that I lost and the new friends that I have gained through this ordeal.

And finally, for me, I think it was a great story, with a happy ending.

CHAPTER 20

Closing

I believe now that I am cured. I am not my old self, but in time I will be. It has been a long, hard battle, one of my toughest yet. It was an experience, it was a challenge, but in the end there is a reward: I get to live. For how long, who knows?

I believe now that I know what life is. We live in a world that is too busy, in a world that is too serious and complicated. You finally buy a car…the one you've always wanted…but in a year it's not good enough anymore, so you have to get a better one, or your house is suddenly too small and you want something bigger. I guess it's alright to want more, but remember to always appreciate what you have. You don't know what you have until you lose it. Not only material things—cherish your family and friends. Every once in a while, give a shout-out and let them know how you feel.

I think there are two kinds of people in this world. You take the proverbial glass of water scenario. That is, half full. Why do people see it as half empty? Why have the negative aspect to everything? Even with a quarter cup—hey, there's still something in there. Why not take the positive outlook towards things? You just might live longer.

Take what you have in life and make it worth everything. Be happy with small things that you have accomplished, and then the bigger things in life will be that much bigger. And then if those don't happen, it won't matter.

Think positively, even in the worst situations, and it will bring positive results.

Read a good book, watch a great movie—something that has meaning to it, like *It's a Wonderful Life*. Have special moments with friends and your family, great experiences, and just know how valuable these moments are in life.

You only live once and, what I say is, I got a second chance. What happens next?!

I would like to leave you with something that was written not by a well-known writer, but by a well-known comedian when he was having a serious moment:

"The paradox in our time in history is that we have taller buildings, but shorter tempers. Wider freeways, but narrower view points. We spend more, but have less. We buy more, but enjoy less. We have bigger houses and smaller families. More conveniences, but less time. We have more degrees, but less sense. More knowledge, but less judgment. More experts, yet more problems. More medicines, but less wellness. We drink too much, smoke too much, spend recklessly, laugh too little, drive too fast, get too angry, stay up too late, get up too tired, read too little, watch TV too much, and pray too seldom.

We have multiplied our possessions, but reduced our values. We talk too much, love too seldom and hate too often. We've learned how to make a living, but not a life. We've added years to our life, but not life to years. We've been to the moon and back, but have trouble crossing the street to meet a new neighbor. We've conquered outer space, but not inner space. We've done larger things, but not better things. We've cleaned up the air, but polluted the soul. We've conquered the atom, but not our prejudice. We write more, but learn less. We plan more, but accomplish less. We've learned to rush, but not to wait. We build more computers to hold more information to produce more copies than ever, but we communicate less and less.

These are the times of fast foods and slow digestions, big men and small character, steep profits and shallow relationships. These are the days of two incomes but more divorce, fancier houses but broken homes. These are the days of quick trips, disposable diapers, throw-away morality, one-night stands, overweight bodies, and pills that do everything from cheer to quiet to kill. It is a time when there is much in the showroom window and nothing in the stockroom. A time when technology can bring this letter to you. A time when you can choose either to share this insight or just hit delete.

Remember to spend some time with your loved ones, because they are not going to be around forever. Remember to say a kind word to someone who looks up to you in awe, because that little person soon will grow up and leave your side. Remember to give a long hug to the one next to you, because that is the only treasure you can give with your heart and it doesn't cost a cent. Remember to say I love you to your partner and your loved ones, but most of all, mean it. A kiss and an embrace will mend hurt when it comes from deep inside of you. Remember to hold hands and cherish the moment, for someday that person will not be there again. Give time to love, give time to speak! And give time to share the precious thoughts in your mind, and always remember: life is not measured by the number of breaths we take, but by the moments that take our breath away."

—George Carlin

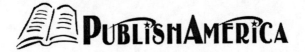

CPSIA information can be obtained at www.ICGtesting.com
Printed in the USA
LVOW130021130613

338231LV00001B/93/P